SO-AEG-866

American Health Care

American Health Care

Realities, Rights, and Reforms

CHARLES J. DOUGHERTY

Theodore Lownik Library
Illinois Benedictine College
Lisle, Illinois 60532

New York   Oxford
OXFORD UNIVERSITY PRESS
1988

362.1
D 732 a

Oxford University Press

Oxford   New York   Toronto
Delhi   Bombay   Calcutta   Madras   Karachi
Petaling Jaya   Singapore   Hong Kong   Tokyo
Nairobi   Dar es Salaam   Cape Town
Melbourne   Auckland

and associated companies in
Beirut   Berlin   Ibadan   Nicosia

Copyright © 1988 by Oxford University Press, Inc.

Published by Oxford University Press, Inc.,
200 Madison Avenue, New York, New York 10016

Oxford is a registered trademark of Oxford University Press

All rights reserved. No part of this publication may be reproduced,
stored in a retrieval system, or transmitted, in any form or by any means,
electronic, mechanical, photocopying, recording, or otherwise,
without the prior permission of Oxford University Press.

Library of Congress Cataloging-in-Publication Data
Dougherty, Charles J.
American health care.
Includes bibliographies and index.
1. Medical care—United States.   2. Medical care—United States—Utilization.
3. Medical policy—United States.   I. Title. [DNLM: 1. Delivery of
Health Care—United States.   2. Health Policy—United States.
3. Public Health Administration—United States.
WA 540 AA1 D73a]
RA395.A3D675   1988   362.1'0973   87-15375
ISBN 0-19-505271-4
ISBN 0-19-505272-2 (pbk.)

9 8 7 6 5 4 3 2 1

Printed in the United States of America
on acid-free paper

for SLD

Preface

This book is an attempt to provide a moral evaluation of American health care. It consists of three main parts: a review and analysis of certain important realities bearing on access to quality health care, a philosophical analysis and defense of the concept of a moral right to health care, and a discussion of various policy alternatives for reform of the system for delivering health care in the United States.

The review in Chapter 1 shows that many Americans, especially among blacks, persons from low-income families, and those with little education, are underserved by the present system. Persons in these groups have significantly worse health characteristics than other Americans. When their greater need for health care is taken into account, they have less access to quality health care than others. They are also among the likeliest groups to be without health insurance. And they are the most probable victims of current efforts to contain spiraling health care costs. These unpleasant American realities set the problem of the book.

Do these persons have a right to health care? If so, to what kinds of care and to how much? These questions are at the center of the philosophical discussions in Chapters 2 through 7. Four contemporary theories of justice and of persons' rights—utilitarianism, egalitarianism, libertarianism, and contractarianism—are examined, and their implications for a right to health care are described. Each theory is then made to play a role in articulating and defending a pluralistically grounded right to health care. This right is the core of four separable rights: to noninterference with one's health, to primary care, to curative care under some circumstances, and to the freedom to buy additional health care not guaranteed by right. From this perspective, it is unjust and a violation of persons' moral rights for the situation described in Chapter 1 to prevail.

What is to be done? This is the central question of Chapters 8, 9, and 10, which examine and evaluate alternative directions for reform of the American system of health care delivery. These include the possibilities of using more of the mechanisms of a free market; of regulating delivery through diagnosis-related groups (DRGs) reimbursement, health maintenance organizations (HMOs), and voucher plans; and of opting for more active government intervention through national health insurance or a national health care service.

Logically, the structure of the work is broadly deductive. Persons have a moral right to health care; many Americans have no ready access to the care to which they have a right; therefore, reforms must be made in the delivery system to ensure that these and all Americans receive the health care to which they have a right. In practice, of course, the empirical complexities of the various alternatives for reform make it impossible to draw simple conclusions about how best to guarantee that the health care rights of all Americans are respected. Nonetheless, tentative suggestions about the directions for reform that are likeliest to bring about this result can be made, and they are offered throughout the discussion of reforms and in the conclusion.

The hope that animates this whole effort is that philosophical reflection can and should make a difference, not only in the lives of individuals, but also in public-policy choices. The book thus addresses three broad professional audiences: philosophers and others concerned with ethics, for whom the conceptual issues surrounding the notion of a moral right to health care are central; social scientists and policy analysts, for whom the facts and theories pertinent to existing and alternative health care delivery systems are key; and health care professionals, who know directly the empirical failings of the American health care system and the realities that these failings bring to persons' lives. If this work can help draw moral theory and health policy closer together and facilitate greater interaction among these three professional groups, it will have justified itself. If it helps in some small way to underscore the moral issues at the center of public-policy debates about health care and its delivery, it will be a success.

Any success that may occur will be due in no small measure to the efforts of the many others whose works I cite and rely on throughout. And this entire project could not have been conceived and executed without the support of Creighton University's sabbatical program. Finally, I am grateful to the many family members, friends, colleagues, and students who have helped me formulate the issues addressed in this study. They are my partners in calling for a more just distribution of health care in the United States.

Omaha   C. J. D.
June 1987

Contents

Realities

1

Some American Health Care Realities

There are many positive things to be said about health care in the United States as the twentieth century draws to a close. In general, the quality of care is high, and access to it is widespread. The nation's health-related statistics are good and generally improving. Life expectancy continues to rise. Infant mortality continues to decline. Government programs and policies, especially Medicare, have met with considerable success and remain highly popular. The poor who are served by the system routinely receive care that is technologically equal to that received by the nonpoor. Rising costs stand out as a problem, but recent steps to control them show signs of having their intended effect. On the whole, then, one may regard the American health care system as a resounding success. But there are also realities that indicate significant failures in the system. Health statistics reveal that blacks and other ethnic minorities, the poor and those with low incomes, and the less educated benefit substantially less from contemporary health care than do other Americans. Figures on access related to need and on health insurance coverage suggest the same conclusion. Health care costs continue to escalate much faster than the rest of the economy, and many of the measures taken and proposed to contain costs have aggravated or likely will aggravate the inequities in delivery of services. These unpleasant realities demand attention.

Access to needed care

Although the infant mortality rate in the United States has continued to decline over the past 35 years from nearly 30 deaths per 1,000 live births in 1950 to approximately 10.6 in 1985, it is still higher than that in many other nations.[1] The rates in Finland, Japan, and Sweden, for example, are between 6.5 and 6.8 per 1,000.[2] Moreoever, the rate of decline in the United States has slowed. Between 1982 and 1984, the rate fell by only 2.7 percent compared with the 4.6 percent average annual decline in the 1970s. Data released in 1985 actually showed an increase in the infant mortality rate in nine states and the District of Columbia. And a good deal of this death rate can be attributed to race, since the rate of deaths among black infants is twice that among whites, and states with large black populations, such as South Carolina, have higher rates of infant deaths (15.7) than do states with small black populations, such as Maine (9.5).[3] Life expectancy at birth displays the same racial dimension. By 1983, the average life span for white females (78.8) was five years longer than that for black females (73.8). White males (71.6) could expect to live more than six years longer than black males (65.2), who on average draw from Social Security retirement income for less than two and one-half months.[4] A report issued by the Department of Health and Human Services (DHHS) in 1985 estimated that more than 60,000 deaths could be prevented annually if mortality rates for blacks and members of other minority groups were as low as the rates for non-Hispanic whites.[5] Eighty percent of these so-called excess deaths occurred in six areas: 18,000 deaths from heart disease and strokes; 11,000 from homicide; 8,100 from cancer; 6,100 from the higher infant mortality rate; 2,150 from cirrhosis; and 1,850 from diabetes. Mortality from lung cancer among black males is 45 percent higher than among white males. Blacks have three times the death rate of whites from cancer of the esophagus and twice that from prostate cancer. Black males under forty-five years of age are ten times more likely to die from hypertension than are white males. Black women have twice the rate of white women of deaths from coronary heart disease. The death rate from cervical cancer among black women is two and one-half times larger than that among white women.

As these death-rate figures suggest, American blacks are also more ill than American whites in general. For example, the rate of tuberculosis in the nonwhite male population over thirty-five years of age is three times that among equivalent whites, and the rate of pelvic inflammatory disease among nonwhite females is two and one-half times the rate among white females.[6] The likelihood of suffering from kidney disease severe enough to require dialysis or transplantation is four times higher among blacks than among whites.[7] American blacks are about six percent more likely than whites to have their activities limited by a chronic health problem (15.4 percent compared with 14.5 percent), and they experience over 46 percent more days per year in bed due to acute or chronic health conditions than do whites (9.5 days per year to 6.5). When they assess their own state of health, an assessment known to be highly correlated with actual state of health, blacks report themselves to be in fair or poor health (18.7 percent) almost 60 percent more frequently than do whites (11.9 percent).[8]

Poverty is highly associated with poor health characteristics. The National Center for Health Statistics estimates that in 1980 more than 29 million Americans, or 14.9 percent of the population, were in the low per capita family-income category, roughly equivalent for most familiy sizes to the federal poverty level.[9] In this group, there is twice as large a percentage of people limited in their activities because of chronic health problems (29.3) as the average for members of families of all incomes (14.5) and over three times the percentage in families with annual incomes of over $25,000 (8.7). Members of low-income families have just under twice as many bed-disability days per year (13.2) as the average for members of all families (6.9) and slightly under three times the amount for members of over-$25,000 families (4.5). When asked to assess their own state of health, people in low-income families rate it poor or fair twice as often (26.6 percent) as members of the financially average families (12.7 percent) and more than four times as often as members of the over $25,000 families (6 percent). There is also evidence that the disparity between the health characteristics of low-income families and high-income families widened from 1970 to 1980. The respective rates of bed-disability days shows this graphically. In 1969, members of low-income families had 1.9 times the annual number of days in bed due to disability as members of the higher income group; but by 1980, the gap had reached 2.3 times. Homeless Americans, whose numbers are rising, must be counted among the poor as well. Estimates of America's homeless population run from 250,000 to 3 million.[10] Compared with the population as a whole, the homeless are three times as likely to assess their health as fair or poor, 50 percent as likely to have disabilities, and nine times as likely to be uninsured for health care.

The health implications of minority racial status and poverty compound each other when they intersect, as they often do. Black Americans are overrepresented among the poor and underrepresented among the wealthy. While blacks constituted 11.8 percent of the United States population in 1980, they made up 25.4 percent of the low-income population and only 5.4 percent of those in families making over $25,000 per capita annually. Thus in proportion to their percentage of the total population, blacks are twice as likely as whites to be poor and half as likely to be wealthy. Consequently, comparisons between the health characteristics of poor blacks and wealthy whites are shocking. Blacks in low-income families are more than two and one-half times as likely (25.5 percent) to be limited in activity due to chronic health problems as are wealthy whites (9 percent). They have almost three and one-half times the rate of bed-disability days per year (15.6 compared with 4.5). And when asked to assess the state of their own health, those who are both black and poor judge it to be fair or poor nearly 30 percent of the time (29.3), while wealthy whites judge their health fair or poor less than 6 percent of the time (5.8).[11] This suggests that the average black person from a low-income family is over five times more likely to have health problems than is the average white person from a high-income family.

If it is fair to assume that blacks from low-income families on average have fewer years of schooling than the average for all families, a third compounding factor is added. Limitation of activity because of chronic health problems is closely associated with education. For all American families, failure to complete twelve years of education, roughly high school, is associated with a 34.9 percent rate of limited activity; for those with sixteen or more years, the equivalent of a college education, the percentage of persons limited by a chronic health problem falls to 11.3. For those with a college education and a high family income, the percentage with chronic health problems that limit activity drops to 9.6; while having no high-school education and a low family income rockets the percentage to 49.2. For bed-disability days, the result is similar. In all families, those without a high-school education average 12.3 days per year in bed with a disabling health condition; those with a college education, 4.8 days. Those with a college education and a high family income have 4 bed-disability days per year, on average; those without a high-school education and from low-income families have 19.7 days. For assessed health status, the effect of education is equally dramatic. In all families, those without a high-school education appraise their health as fair or poor 32.8 percent of the time; while those who attended college do so only 5.7 percent of the time—a factor of more than five and one-half. The combination of a college education and high family income yields just 4.2 percent who claim fair or poor health status, whereas the combination of no high-school education and low family income yields a whopping 46 percent.[12] Given the general reliability of these assessments, this means that the poorest and the least educated Americans are ten times more likely to have health problems than are the wealthiest and the best educated Americans. The rates of visual, hearing, speech, paralysis, and orthopedic impairments is, almost without exception, substantially higher among families that are nonwhite, low income, and less educated.[13]

In terms of health outcomes, these statistics suggest that American blacks, people with low or poverty-level incomes, and the less educated fare worst in the United States. The human realities behind these figures are multiple personal tragedies of "excess death" and the unnecessary pain, suffering, and disability found disproportionately among members of these groups. It is more difficult to determine just what accounts for these disparities. Some of the causes may say more about American society in general than about the health care system in particular. In spite of considerable strides since the 1960s, de facto racism is still a significant feature of American life. Blacks are among the poorest and least educated, and therefore among the least healthy, of Americans. Many of the disadvantaged are served by Medicare, Medicaid, and other government programs, and many hospitals and other providers absorb the costs of charity care and unpaid debts. But in general, health care and the health insurance on which it often depends are distributed in the same way that most goods and services are distributed in the United States: largely on a pay-as-you-go basis. This marketplace mode of distribution is bound by its nature to work against the interests of those least well-off financially. Furthermore, there is a clear link between health and poverty in American society: being unable to work because of disability is a potent source of poverty itself. And a relative lack of education certainly tends to promote poor understanding of preventive health care as well as less sophistication in drawing appropriate and timely benefits from the health care system.

But it is also known that access to health care can make a difference in health outcomes.[14] Although life expectancy and infant mortality have increased and decreased respectively for the past thirty-five years for Americans, the rates of improvement accelerated after the establishment of Medicare and Medicaid in the mid-1960s, as these programs expanded access to care for many of the elderly and the poor. For black Americans, visits to physicians increased by 33 percent between 1964 and 1976, from 3.6 visits per person per year to 4.8. In this same period, life expectancy increased by about two years for all white Americans and about three years for blacks. Infant mortality declined from about 22 to about 14 deaths per 1,000 births for all Americans, and from about 35 to about 25 deaths per 1,000 births for blacks. It is only reasonable to suppose that increased access to health care helped bring about these improvements. There is little question, for example, that publicly funded health centers placed in areas of high poverty and minority population saved lives by contributing to a decline in infant mortality.[15] Recently, it has been estimated that health outcomes are so associated with greater use of health care facilities that a 10 percent increase in per capita health expenditures would decrease death rates by another 1.57 percent. By contrast, when California dropped more than 250,000 people from its Medicaid (Medi-Cal) program in 1982, the number of these individuals who could identify a usual source of care fell from 96 percent to 50 percent, those extremely or very satisfied with their health care went from 91 percent to 60 percent, and those convinced they could get the care they needed went from 83 percent to 38 percent. Worse yet, researchers documented "clinically meaningful deterioration" in the health of members of this group, including a loss of blood-pressure control among hypertensives. And a follow-up study has confirmed the long-term negative health effects among those cut off from MediCal benefits.[16]

Over the past several decades, access to health care in general has improved dramatically indeed. From the mid-1950s to the early 1980s, the percentage of nonwhites visiting a physician at least once a year rose from about 50 to over 80, nearly equal to the rate for all whites.[17] The visits per family in 1980 were 4.8 for all white families and 4.5 for all black families.[18] The percentage of low-income persons seeing a physician once a year went from about 55 in 1953 to about 80 in 1982.[19] By 1980, the number of visits per year was actually more for members of low-income families (5.9) than for all families (4.7).[20] In the same year, the number of visits by blacks from low-income families (6 per year) exceeded the number by whites from high-income families (4.6).[21] And Medicare facilitated a substantial increase in hospital access by the elderly: a 25 percent increase in use by this group occurred immediately after the program went into effect.[22] There seems little question that Medicare has prolonged the average life span of the elderly and enhanced the quality of their lives.

If improvements in health characteristics are associated with increases in access to care and significant improvements have been made since the 1950s in promoting access to care, why are the health characteristics of some groups of Americans still so poor compared with those of others?

Part of the answer probably has to do with the changed nature of poverty in the United States. In the early decades of this century, poverty was a mass phenomenon; today, it is a marginal one. As such, it has become more highly focused on fewer persons and more closely associated with the compounding factors of race and less education. It is also closely connected with high rates of unemployment, some of which is directly attributable to health problems and disabilities. The plight of the worst off in an affluent society thus appears countercyclical: the better conditions are for most people, the worse they are relatively for those excluded from that affluence.[23] This is especially clear in the association of poverty and health conditions. When a large proportion of the population is poor and unemployed or underemployed, it will normally include many people of good or average health. But when poverty becomes a marginal phenomenon, health problems will be overrepresented among them. At least this appears true of recent American experience.

Simply put, the health care needs of nonwhites, the poor, and the less educated are generally greater than average, perhaps significantly so. If this is the case, then achieving a rough equality of access between black and white, poor and nonpoor, and less and more educated will not result in equal health outcomes. But if the point of health care is to prevent premature death and unnecessary pain, suffering, and disability, then equality of results is what matters. Thus the more deprived groups need more care, maybe much more, if results are to be made more equal. But they are not now getting the greater care they need. Using the number of bed-disability days as an index of need, for example, data from the late 1970s show that in groups with similar medical needs, high-income persons visited physicians 73 percent more often than low-income persons.[24] And among those assessing their health as fair or poor, whites visited physicians more often than blacks among the poor (10 percent more), among the near poor (14 percent more), and among the nonpoor (26 percent more).[25] Compared with those who are poor, black, and in fair or poor health, those who are not poor, white, but also in fair or poor health saw physicians 50 percent more often. Thus judged in relationship to need, black and low-income Americans are not yet close to enjoying equal access to health care.

Some of the reasons for this are easy to see. Even though the supply of physicians is increasing, the Department of Health and Human Services estimated in 1982 that over 16 million Americans live in areas of the nation where there is a shortage of physicians.[26] Many of these regions are heavily populated by just the groups in question here: their poverty and race does not attract physicians who must establish a practice and retire medical-school debts and who are also overwhelmingly white. For example, it was reported in 1980 that fifty-one of Mississippi's eighty-two counties had no obstetrician and fifty had no pediatrician.[27] And the lack of physicians serving the inner-city black population is equally notorious. The number of physicians in Chicago dropped from 1 per 1,000 population to 1 per 4,000 from 1950 to 1970, while the number in the city's suburbs went up correspondingly.[28] In 1983, it was reported that 24.5 million Americans (10.8 percent of the population) had no regular source of health care. This figure included 10.4 percent of the white population, but 13.5 percent of blacks; 10.5 percent of the nonpoor, but 11.9 percent of the poor; and 9.7 percent of college graduates, but 12.4 percent of those with less than a high-school education. Just short of 4 million families claimed to have needed health care that they did not obtain, the percentage of poor families deferring care (8.9) being more than twice that of nonpoor families (4.4). And a shocking 1 million families reported that they were refused care for financial reasons. As one might expect, the rate for poor families turned away from the health care system was two and one-half times larger (2.8 percent) than that for nonpoor families (1.1 percent). Hispanics, poor and nonpoor, reported being turned away more than twice as often (3.3 percent) as blacks (1.5 percent) and whites (1.4 percent).[29]

This large gap in access to health care indicates a failure in the Medicaid program, which was begun in the mid-1960s as a welfare program designed to make health care available to the nation's poor. But unlike its legislative companion, Medicare—which establishes federal guidelines for universal enrollment of Americans who are over sixty-five, those who have permanent disabilities, and those who suffer from end-stage renal failure—Medicaid eligibility is established by each state. The federal government's commitment is financial, paying a percentage of each state's program costs. This makes for a nationally fragmented effort to care for the poor.[30] Because most states tie eligibility to Aid for Families with Dependent Children (AFDC) standards, poor single persons, poor couples without children, and poor families with both parents at home are generally ineligible for support. Furthermore, although some states are relatively generous in their eligibility standards, many states set the standard for Medicaid considerably below federal poverty guidelines. On average, states cover about 35 percent of their low-income population with Medicaid, ranging from a high of 46 percent in Massachusetts to a low of 14 percent in South Dakota.[31] The result is that millions of poor Americans cannot afford to pay for their own health care but do not qualify for Medicaid: some 60 percent of America's poor are not eligible for Medicaid.[32] In 1981, there were federal cuts in both the Medicaid and the AFDC programs that further disadvantaged the already disadvantaged. In one poor Boston community, for example, from January 1980 to June 1982, 18 percent fewer families were receiving AFDC payments, Medicaid-covered visits to local health centers went down by 25 percent, the number of women receiving inadequate prenatal care rose by an estimated 60 percent, and the infant mortality rate increased by 53 percent.[33] In each of the five years after 1981, the government reduced Medicare and Medicaid spending by diminishing payments to hospitals, physicians, and states.[34]

In addition, much of Medicaid's annual budget does not go to the nation's poor in the senses that Congress probably intended and the public probably expects. Instead, in 1980 approximately 66 percent of all Medicaid payments went to the aged and disabled, essentially supplementing gaps in the Medicare program, and 40 percent of Medicaid's outlays went to pay for the long-term nursing care of elderly Americans.[35] As much as 70 percent of all nursing care is paid for by Medicaid because although the need is focused in the population over sixty-five years of age, Medicare does not cover custodial care and the private insurance industry has not marketed an affordable policy to the general public.[36] This use of Medicaid money does serve a needy population, to be sure, but it also means that most of the program's budget does not go where it is widely thought to go: to provide health care to those who are poor for most or all of their lives.

Finally, the program is hobbled by the large number of physicians who do not treat Medicaid patients. In 1982, over 21 percent of all primary-care physicians (general practice, general surgery, internal medicine, obstetrics and gynecology, and pediatrics) did not participate in the program. Among medical specialists, 32 percent did not participate. More than 15 percent of surgical specialists were nonparticipants. And just short of 40 percent of all psychiatrists and cardiologists treated no Medicaid patients.[37] But 15.8 percent of all primary-care physicians have large Medicaid practices, in which 30 percent or more of the patients are on Medicaid. Although there is no evidence of widespread abuse, there are suspicious statistical characteristics among physicians who run large Medicaid practices. Compared with their peers in other practices, these physicians are significantly less board certified (26 percent compared with 43 percent), twice as likely to be graduates of foreign medical schools, and, in the very large Medicaid practices, much more likely to be general practitioners over sixty years old.[38] Thus Medicaid guarantees the poor access neither to health care nor, when it is provided, to the kind of doctors who serve most other Americans.

Nor is the problem of access solved by private health insurance. In fact, the number of uninsured Americans increased from 29 million in 1979 to 35 million by the mid-1980s.[39] This substantial increase is partly accounted for by an increase in unemployment early in this period, since most Americans receive health insurance through their place of employment. The unemployed were four times (28.6 percent) as likely to be uninsured as the employed (7.1 percent) in 1982. But employment does not guarantee health insurance because many of the self-employed, temporary and part-time workers, and those working in small businesses and for low wages are often uninsured or underinsured. Moreover, in 1982 19.3 percent of adult Americans were not in the labor force, and 7.9 percent of them were reported to be uninsured. And the pattern of the least well-off repeats itself in insurance coverage, with one exception. Blacks were 67 percent more likely to be uninsured (11.9 percent) than whites (7.1 percent), and Hispanics were more than twice as likely to be uninsured (14.5 percent). Members of poor families were four times more likely to be uninsured (20.1 percent) than members of nonpoor families (5 percent). The likelihood of having health insurance rose with the level of education from 13.5 percent uninsured among those without a high-school education to 5.4 percent among those with a college education. The exception is people in the age group of nineteen to twenty-four, which was the most uninsured and underinsured of all age groups.[40] A 1977 survey found 16 percent of these young adults uninsured for the whole year and another 14.3 percent uninsured for a part of the year, for a total annual uninsured rate of 30.3 percent.[41] And a 1985 report showed that insurance coverage is not matched to the apparent need for it. Of persons limited in activity by chronic health problems, those from families with low per capita incomes were twice as likely to be uninsured

(20.5 percent) as those from high-income families (10 percent). The poor and uninsured had nearly three times the number of bed-disability days per year (13.3 days) as the high-income insured (4.5 days). And of those who assessed their health as fair or poor, three times as many of the low-income family members (23.4 percent) as the high-income family members (7.2 percent) were uninsured.[42]

Whether one falls into one of these groups of the uninsured through age, unemployment, or employment with a business that provides neither group coverage nor the wages needed to purchase individual coverage appears to be a matter of luck—bad luck.[43] Being uninsured not only increases anxiety for those aware of its significance, but also deters people from seeking health care when it is needed. In the late 1970s, insured patients made physician visits 54 percent more often than the uninsured, and they received 90 percent more hospital care.[44] Some of this differential may be self-selected; that is, the uninsured are likely to refrain from turning to the health care system when they know that they cannot afford to pay directly for the care they need. In some cases, there is frank refusal by providers to care for the uninsured who are unable to demonstrate the ability to pay.[45] In other cases, the refusal is less frank but still dangerous. A study at Cook County Hospital (Ill.) of "dumping"—that is, transferring patients from private hospitals to public hospitals—revealed that 87 percent of those transferred were dumped because they had inadequate health insurance; 89 percent were black or Hispanic, and 81 percent were unemployed.[46] Only 6 percent of these patients gave written consent for the transfer, and 24 percent were in unstable clinical condition at the transferring hospital. The mean treatment delay caused by these transfers was over five hours, with the predictable result that the death rate among the transferred patients (9.4 percent) was increased—increased, in fact, to over twice the rate among nontransferred patients (3.8 percent).

While no one can justify the behavior of those private hospitals that jeopardize uninsured patients' lives by dumping them on the public system, providing health care to the poor who are not covered by Medicaid and not covered adequately by private insurance can be a substantial financial burden on hospitals. In 1982, an estimated 22.5 million Americans fell into this category and depended wholly or largely on charity for their health care.[47] It cost private hospitals about $3.2 billion in 1982, while state and local governments spent about $9.5 billion in grants and appropriations to cover costs related to nonreimbursed care at public hospitals. The American Hospital Association (AHA) estimates that in 1984, its member hospitals furnished a total of $5.7 billion in uncompensated care, an increase from $2.8 billion in 1980.[48] This situation is worsening in part because of changes in the federal government's system for reimbursing hospital Medicare costs

(DRGs) and in part because of a general demand that rising hospital costs be contained. The federal Health Care Financing Administration (HCFA) had refused, for example, to reimburse hospitals that serve large numbers of poor Medicare patients at higher rates than other hospitals, even though these patients, both elderly and poor, are generally more expensive to care for than other patients because they are often more severely ill and take longer to place in nursing homes.[49] Public and private demands for hospital cost containment have led many hospitals to restrict entry by those who are uninsured and unlikely to pay, since the cost of their care must be absorbed by higher prices elsewhere. Between 1980 and 1982, for example, the number of persons both poor and inadequately covered by health insurance rose by a dramatic 20.9 percent, but free care provided by both public and private hospitals rose by only 3.8 percent.[50] These trends not only are a sign of a failure in the American health care system, but also suggest that many persons working in that system, including health care professionals, have been involved in explicit planning to limit or outright deny health care to those who cannot demonstrate the ability to pay for it. This is probably a morally unsettling problem for many of these individuals and is certainly a bad situation generally for the ethos of the health care professions.

Quality of care

Gaps in Medicaid, in insurance coverage, and in charity care may therefore create barriers to more complete access in terms of need for low-income Americans who are also disproportionately black and poorly educated. This may account for some of their relatively poor health characteristics. But the fact that these poor health characteristics are present in the face of increased and virtually equal access, in some cases more access, to health care by blacks and by low-income families suggests another problem. They may indeed have access to health care, but it may be to health care of an inferior quality.

One of the best ways to ensure a high quality of health care—that is, appropriate, timely, comprehensive, and continual care—is to ensure access to primary care. The widespread ability to identify a primary-care physician as the usual source of health care and to have access to that physician in his or her office are structural marks of quality health care. In order for this to be accomplished, there must be a great number of primary-care physicians spread throughout the patient population. In industrial democracies other than the United States, this is more or less the case. In Western Europe, Canada, Japan, Australia, and New Zealand, 40 to 50 percent of all clinical physicians are general practitioners.[51] There is an explicit commitment to universal access to primary care in physicians' offices, with specialists (generally the salaried staff of hospitals) available on their referral. In the United States, by contrast, only 15 percent of clinical physicians are general practitioners, and, as is already evident, there is no guarantee of universal access to them. This may account in part for the fact that although the United States has a higher standard of living than most of these other nations, all of them have longer life expectancy and lower infant mortality rates.

When primary care is unavailable or difficult to obtain, the hospital becomes the locus of health care. The hospital is frequently an inappropriate and overly expensive setting for the treatment of health problems, many of which could have been avoided or lessened in severity had they been diagnosed and treated in a timely manner in a physician's office. Blacks, the poor, and the less educated show up disproportionately in hospital outpatient departments and in emergency rooms (ERs). When asked in the late 1970s to name the site of their last encounter with a physician, 84 percent of white respondents said a physician's office, but only 64 percent of blacks did. Among those who said a hospital emergency room, 20 percent were black and only 8 percent were white. And those with incomes of less than $5,000 per year were more than twice as likely (15 percent) as those making more than $15,000 (7 percent) to have met a physician in the ER. Data from 1982 indicate that only 3 percent of higher income, insured urban whites considered a hospital ER to be their usual source of care, while 36 percent of poor, uninsured urban blacks did. And studies show that in the early 1980s, 82 percent of the white patients who entered hospitals were admitted by private physicians, but only 65 percent of blacks who entered hospitals were. The fact that such a large percentage of black and poor Americans have no primary care, but rely on hospitals, suggests that they will be cared for later than is appropriate, when their conditions are more acute and less responsive to treatment. There are data to support this. The cancers of white Americans are detected earlier than those of blacks, and the cancers of paying patients are found earlier than those of the nonpaying.[52] Early detection of cancer can, of course, make a significant difference in the outcome of the disease, and these differences of diagnosis may help to account for some of the dramatically higher death rates from cancer among black Americans. Emergency-room care not only is less timely than primary care in a physician's office, but also is less continual and comprehensive. The significant reliance of blacks on less effective hospital care may therefore help to explain the much higher rate of kidney failure due to uncontrolled hypertension among blacks. It is simply not often enough detected and managed properly with the help of a primary-care physician.[53]

The quality of care can also be affected by racial and cultural barriers, especially when the provider and the patient have differing backgrounds, understandings, and expectations. There are, for example, ethnic and racial differences in appraising the nature and significance of disease.[54] Unawareness or insensitivity to these differences on the part of providers can lead to misunderstandings, noncompliance, and less than effective health care. And the hospital ER is not the best setting to bridge cultural and racial distances. In one study of cases of myocardial infarction in an ER, for example, it was shown that white patients tended to describe their symptoms differently from black patients.[55] This difference may increase the hazard of misdiagnosis among the latter, since so many black Americans rely on the hospital ER but only about 2 percent of all physicians in America are black.[56] Communication difficulties can be further compounded because many of the physicians who treat the poor and the racial and ethnic minorities in America's inner cities are themselves graduates of foreign medical schools who often have problems with the English language. In one poor section of Brooklyn, New York, for example, the staff of a municipal hospital is 97 percent foreign-educated physicians.[57] And some have expressed the concern that one of the roles that the poor, black, and less educated play in America's teaching hospitals, the role of "teaching material" for medical students and residents, may build racial and class prejudices into the socialization of American physicians. The use of these patients to hone medical skills that will then be applied largely, even exclusively, for the benefit of private patients in white suburbs may indirectly teach contempt for the disadvantaged and further diminish the quality of their health care.[58] Ironically, in teaching hospitals and in the large public hospitals, poor, black, and less educated patients may be receiving health care, even too much health care, that from a technological point of view is equal to the best anywhere. Yet the inferior interpersonal character of their care may still diminish its overall quality.[59] This probably contributes to the substantially higher level of dissatisfaction these groups report regarding their health care.[60] Because the human dimensions of the way a person is treated no doubt affects that person's readiness to use a social system and to comply with its prescriptions, the lack of quality health care for America's disadvantaged may account for part of their poor health characteristics.

Rising costs

The rising costs of health care and some of the changing financial pressures in the system require attention both in themselves and because they may tend to aggravate the circumstances of the medically needy and those already poorly served by the system. Per capita spending on health care in the United States has increased (in constant 1982 dollars) from $503 in 1950 to $776 in 1965 to over $1,365 by the early 1980s.[61] This represented 4.4 percent of the gross national product (GNP) in 1950, 6.1 percent in 1965, and 10.6 percent by 1984.[62] From 1970 to 1984, costs increased at an average of 12.6 percent annually. Although the rate of increase has begun to slow (9.1 percent in 1984, about 7.5 percent in 1986), the rate of inflation in health care is still around twice the rate of inflation in the rest of the economy. The Department of Health and Human Services projects that even at a slower rate of increase, the total spent on health care in the United States could reach $600 billion in 1990, 11.3 percent of the GNP.[63]

The federal government has many health care–related expenditures, but the major federal health care commitments are the Medicare and Medicaid programs, which together accounted for 90 percent of federal health care spending and about 10 percent of the total 1984 federal budget.[64] As a percentage of total health care spending in the United States, the federal share is about 29; state and local governments' share is about 12. Thus approximately 41 percent of national spending on health care is paid for publicly. This is up from 26 percent in 1965; and the percentage paid from private sources, including insurance, decreased from 74 in 1965 to 59 in 1984. Although an apparently large public commitment by American standards, it is not so large as other nations' health care investment per capita. The 1980 per capita public expenditure on health was $439, compared with $571 on education and $632 on defense. Worldwide, this ranked the United States eighth in per capita defense spending, sixteenth in education, and thirteenth in health. Compared with Western Europe and Canada in the mid-1970s, the United States financed the least of its health care expenditures publicly and the most privately.[65]

The federal government spent $20 billion in Medicaid and $61 billion on Medicare in 1984; the latter had risen to almost $74 billion by 1986.[66] The Congressional Budget Office (CBO) projects that the total cost of these programs will almost double by 1990, to reach $152 billion. If this projection is accurate and Medicare expenditures grow to the projected $119 billion by 1990, at the same rates of income, the CBO predicts bankruptcy of the trust fund that finances Medicare sometime in the 1990s. The government's response has been to increase patients' cost-sharing in Medicare and to introduce in the program a more restrictive, prospective method of reimbursing hospitals for the care of Medicare patients (DRGs). Although these changes have raised concern that the elderly and others covered by Medicare will suffer, they have probably helped to bring about a drop in the utilization rate of hospitals and a decline in the average length of stay (LOS). From 1981 to 1984, nonelderly admissions to hospitals decreased by 10 percent, and the nonelderly LOS dropped by about 7 percent, from 5.9 days to 5.5 days.[67] Among the elderly population covered by Medicare, although hospital admissions have dropped only slightly, LOS has dropped more than twice as much as among the nonelderly, from 10.4 days to 8.8 days, or about 15 percent. This suggests first that the nonelderly may have more discretion in their use of hospitals, but second that the elderly are being released from needed hospitalization considerably quicker than in the recent past. Since the United States already has the shortest hospital LOS of any comparable nation, further pressure for early hospital discharge may be dangerous to the elderly. Furthermore, these declines in hospital admissions and LOS have not been accompanied by any drop in the increase of the cost-per-patient of each day in a hospital, so whatever savings may be realized from these changes appear to be due to using the health care system less and not from using it more efficiently.

Rising costs have affected the poor as well. They have found the eligibility criteria for Medicaid made more restrictive and other programs targeted toward them dismantled; such programs included the National Health Services Corps, which had provided support for medical-school tuition in return for years of service in high poverty and medically underserved areas.[68] Beside the obvious barrier that these cuts create for access to a group already disadvantaged, there is a double injustice that derives from recent tax policies. At the same time that their Medicaid benefits were cut in 1981, the poor were subjected to a tax increase, while all other Americans had their tax burden lowered.[69] In 1979, a family of four at the poverty line paid 1.9 percent of its income in federal taxes. By 1985, the federal tax on that same family had risen to 10.4 percent of its income. While federal income tax payments as a share of pretax income fell for the rest of the nation, the share for the poorest 20 percent of the nation rose from 0.5 percent of pretax income to 1.2 percent, more than doubling. At the same time, federal tax subsidies for health care costs to employers and employees in the form of tax exclusions for the former and medical-expense deductions for the latter outstripped in value the amount of funds committed by the federal government to Medicaid.[70] In 1980, the federal government spent $12.7 billion on Medicaid, but the value of the tax benefits provided by exclusions and deductions totaled $20.2 billion. Since these tax benefits go overwhelmingly to businesses and to higher income Americans, and since Medicaid goes to the poor and to those made poor by the costs of custodial care, the conclusion that the federal government invests more public or would-be public resources on health care for the wealthy and less on health care for the poor appears both inescapable and morally wrong.[71]

Pressure to contain costs is also coming from private industry, and this may help to account for some of the drop in nonelderly hospital admissions.

From 1977 to 1982, annual health insurance payments by companies rose nationally from $33 billion to $78 billion.[72] Goodyear, for example, spent over $165 million on employee health care in 1983. In that same year, the average health care payment per employee in 850 large and mid-sized companies was between $2,100 and $2,400, having risen through the late 1970s from 20 to 30 percent annually. Of the total American spending on health care, business pays about 33 percent. Since over 40 percent of this investment is paid for hospital charges, businesses have begun to restrict their employees' access to hospitals. A survey of a 1,000 American corporations in 1985 revealed that 63 percent required employees to pay a deductible before the company would begin paying their hospital bills, compared with only 30 percent of corporations that had imposed deductibles just three years earlier.[73] Between 1982 and 1984, Business Roundtable Companies increased their employee health plan premiums by an average of 47.7 percent, their deductibles by 85.2 percent, and their co-payments by 96.4 percent.[74] Other cost-containing measures are being used: mandatory second opinions before surgery, preadmission certification before hospitalization, restriction of employees to certain providers who agree to control costs, mandatory use of outpatient services, and retrospective review of hospital charges. These measures will likely help to save money, but their effects on employees' access to quality health care and on their health itself remain to be seen. Of special concern is the impact of cost-sharing measures on low-income wage earners and on the working poor.

To a great extent, the whole health care system is becoming more of a business itself. Under the pressure of cost controls by the public and private sectors, American health care is becoming more commercialized, more competitive, more marketing oriented. As hospitals have become less the charitable institutions they once were, they have benefited less from charity. Philanthropy, once a large portion of hospitals' operating budgets, has dwindled to a pittance.[75] Capital for hospitals is now raised by the sale of tax-exempt bonds in the case of not-for-profit hospitals and through the stock market in the case of for-profit hospitals. The hospital phenomenon of the 1980s is the investor owned for-profit (IOFP) hospital chain. Between 1977 and 1982, the number of hospitals owned and managed by the IOFPs increased by 42 percent, their total number of beds growing by 62 percent.[76] By 1984, they owned or managed 15 percent of all nongovernment acute general-hospital beds in the United States, and 50 percent of the nongovernment psychiatric beds. Twenty-five percent of all health maintenance organizations (HMOs) are now run for profit,[77] as are a great number of preferred provider organizations, free-standing emergicenters and surgicenters, and home health care companies. Advertising and promotion of health care and health care–related services now abound, coming from for-profit and not-for-profit institutions alike. And although physicians' income had its first modern decline in 1983,[78] physicians are still the highest paid of any occupational group, making five times the average American worker's income.[79] Fees for physicians' services increased ninefold from the start of Medicare and Medicaid in 1965 to 1985, by which time they accounted for 19 percent of national health care expenditures.[80] It is difficult to fully and fairly appraise the impact of these large cultural trends, but it is only reasonable to suppose that as American health care becomes more and more a business and less and less a community service, those groups already disadvantaged in the American business environment will be further disadvantaged. One can expect to find the poor, blacks, and the less well educated disproportionately represented among them.

Rights

2

A Right to Health Care

One of the most straightforward ways to focus the moral issues suggested by the health care inequities described in Chapter 1 is to consider the concept of a right. Do all Americans have a right to health care? If the answer is yes, many other questions immediately follow. To what kinds of health care do Americans have a right? To how much care do they have a right? Who is duty bound to provide this care? How is it to be delivered and paid for? Although each of these questions is important, the most fundamental one is the first. Unless this question is answered affirmatively, the other questions must be dropped or substantially rephrased—that is, asked in such a way as to make no appeal to the concept of a right. In order to see if this question can be answered affirmatively, the nature of a right must be explored and some plausible connections between rights and health care established.

The concept of a right

Contemporary Americans are familiar   some would say too familiar—with claims about rights. We follow international issues concerning assertions about human rights and domestic constitutional battles about the right to privacy and the right to life. We may find ourselves insisting on or yielding the right of way at traffic intersections and debating the relative merits of claims about smokers' and nonsmokers' rights. From the assertions of nations to self-determination to the demands of grandparents to visit their grandchildren, Americans' political and personal experience is filled with claims about rights. To twentieth-century Americans, the language of rights seems a most natural way to articulate and emphasize those demands that claimants regard as important moral demands. This observation reveals a first important feature of rights. To focus an issue as one bearing on rights is to insist on its seriousness by relating the issue to that which one claims to be entitled. The claim of right is thus a claim of entitlement.[1] The claim of a right to free political speech, for example, is an insistence on the seriousness of a citizen's entitlement to freedom from interference with public comment and criticism.

Although our most serious entitlements, such as freedom of speech and religion, are often claimed in terms of rights, it is important to realize that the entitlement itself often creates the seriousness of the claim, and not simply the substance of the thing that is claimed. An example may help make this point. Suppose that Smith is waiting on line at the post office, the next person to be served. If Jones comes in later but tries to be served first, Smith might justly claim the right to go next. Given the social rules of lining up, Smith is entitled to be served in the order in which she entered the line. Obviously, this is not an issue of great moment, but that is just the point. Smith is entitled to be next, and this entitlement lends seriousness to her claim.

Even if we add a serious moral claim on Jones's side, the same result emerges in terms of rights, although perhaps a different moral situation is created in general. Suppose that Jones insists on being served before Smith because he has left a sick infant waiting in a car, and suppose further that there is no special pressure on Smith's own schedule. Probably we would say that Smith still has the right to go next, even though it would certainly be a good thing for Smith to give up her right for the sake of Jones's infant. Here the seriousness is on Jones's side, but the right is still Smith's to claim or relinquish. And in both cases, whether serious or not, should Smith choose to insist on the right to be served next, it is reasonable to expect that the clerk or the postmaster will uphold Smith's entitlement. Of course, it is also reasonable to expect that the vindication of Smith's right will be accompanied by overt signs of moral disapproval in the case involving Jones's sick infant. As important as they are, rights are not the only important moral dimension of a situation.

Other key features of rights can be drawn from this mundane example. The entitlement to be served according to one's place in line follows from the existence of a social rule governing the manner of serving the public in a post office, a bank, or anywhere else that the practice of forming lines prevails. Sometimes the social rule is ambiguous, as at a bus stop where people may or may not form a line and therefore there may or may not be a right to enter the bus in a certain order. Sometimes it is tacit, as at a grocery counter where a line appears to form but no one is certain who may be next. Sometimes it is an explicit social rule, as printed on the sign at a bank indicating how the line is to form. Sometimes it is both explicit and formal, as in taking a number to ensure orderly service at a bakery. The point to notice in these cases is that the having of a right depends on the existence of a social rule. When forced to justify a claim to a right, appeal can be made first to the rule that gives the right its meaning. The existence of the rule itself depends on the roles that people play in the larger social network of cultural practices and formal institutions.[2] And as the variety of these cases suggests, it is not always obvious whether a right exists because it is not always easy to identify the rules and roles from which the right may follow.

Reference to social rules suggests an important distinction that bears on rights and claims about them. By a right, we sometimes mean a legal right; sometimes, a moral right. With legal rights, the social rules on which the right depends are explicit laws or judicial precedents. If a traffic accident occurs because one driver failed to yield the right of way to another, a law was broken. If an employee is passed over for a promotion for which he or she was next in line by virtue of company policy or union contract, a court may vindicate that employee's right to the promotion as a matter of law. The second driver and the passed-over employee have legal rights that follow from relatively explicit legislative and judicial acts. But in the cases sketched above, the rights are largely moral rights because they follow from rules and practices with a largely moral standing. That the next person in line at the post office is served next is a morally plausible rule, but probably not a law.

Although it is often difficult to determine the controlling law or judicial precedent in a given situation, generally it is much more difficult to isolate moral rules. Compared with written laws and court decisions, moral rules are usually tacit and vague. But in spite of its difficulty, identification of moral rights and the moral rules on which they are based is quite an important task for two reasons. First, since morality is composed of the good and bad, the right and wrong of everyday life, we find ourselves more often in situations in which a person's moral rights are at issue than in situations in which the issue is primarily legal. In many questions of fairness, for example, moral rights are probably at stake. Second, our ability to make, criticize, and change laws depends in part on our abilty to recognize that some laws and proposed laws embody, and some violate, moral rules. In other words, questions of morality and moral rights are both more pervasive and more fundamental than are questions of legality and legal rights.

Another element apparent in this example is the enforceability of rights. To have a right effectively is to have a social guarantee against the standard threats to the enjoyment of the right.[3] Smith's right to be served next at the post office will amount to little unless the postal clerk and the others waiting in line acknowledge this right and feel bound to act on it in general. This acknowledgment need not be explicit or conscious. In usual situations, it will suffice that the clerk serve Smith in proper order and that others line up behind Smith. But when a right is challenged or violated, conscious acknowledgment of the right must be made and social sanction imposed against violators. Sanctions vary with the nature of the right and the gravity of its violation. Causing a traffic accident by violating a right will result in a fine and perhaps in imprisonment. Moving ahead of someone at the grocery-counter line may result in only nonverbal condemnation. The point remains, however, that there must be means by which rightful entitlements are routinely guaranteed. Rights derive their practical force from the obligations of nonclaimants to respect them. Put another way, when a right exists for one person, some other person or persons have a corresponding duty to acknowledge and act on that right. Rights and duties, with some exceptions, are correlative: rights entail duties and vice versa.[4]

The case in the post office also shows that the possessor of the right may exercise or relinquish the right. Smith can allow Jones or anyone else to go ahead, even though she also has the right to refuse to allow them to do so. This may be done for any number of reasons or for no specific reason: to be gracious, to repay a kindness, merely to be spontaneous. Or it may be done under the weight of very important moral considerations, such as the case of Jones's sick infant waiting in the car. If Smith is next, she has the right to be served next, but this right does not exhaust the moral dimensions of the situation. In other words, it may sometimes not be good to insist on one's rights—not good for others, but also not good for the bearer of the right. Clearly, for Smith to insist on the right to go next is not good for the Jones's baby. But it may also not be good for Smith's own personality—not good to fix so exclusively on what she is entitled to, no matter what the consequences for others.

Not only may the possessor of a right be in a position to relinquish the exercise of it, but there may be situations in which another person may be justified in overriding the right, either because another right takes precedence or because of an extreme set of circumstances. In other words, although a right usually establishes the entitlement of an individual, it is not morally absolute. Instead, rights are prima facie entitlements, entitlements normally binding unless something of substantially greater moral significance overrules them. Smith may have the right to go next at a traffic intersection, for example, but a police car or an emergency vehicle may "trump" her right with another superseding and legally recognized right. And extreme cases may void or suspend enforcement of many rights. Imagine a gunman demanding to go ahead of Smith on the post-office line and threatening to take lives if not served next. Although Smith still has the moral right to be served next, it would be wrong for Smith and the postal clerk to insist on that right at the risk of endangering others. The gravity of the situation overrules the enforcement of Smith's right. So although rights are ordinarily prior to other moral considerations, they are not always so. When they are not will be hard to determine in advance of the facts. Except for cases of legally defined priorities of rights (emergency vehicles first, for example), there are no rules governing the suspension of rules. In circumstances of genuine catastrophe, for instance, the normal rules of social interaction are overwhelmed by events and with them the prevalence of normal moral rights. Still, short of trumping by a stronger right or of catastrophe, a strong presumption must rest with the priority of moral rights.

Another important distinction can be explored in the example. Many theorists have distinguished between negative and positive rights.[5] Broadly, a negative right is a liberty right, a right to be protected from interference with a freedom of thought or action. A positive right is an access right, a right to be provided with necessary goods and services. Most of the rights generally deferred to in American experience are negative rights: freedom from governmental interference with political speech, religious belief, assembling with others for lawful purposes, and so on. These are traditional rights in American society, and in theory they cost little, only forebearance. The right to an education, to housing, or to health care, by contrast, would be positive rights. Americans are far more ambiguous in their assent to these rights, and they certainly do cost. Although often useful, this broad distinction may not always apply or may apply, but not so neatly as might be supposed. In the post-office line, for example, Smith's right to be served in the order in which she entered the line is both positive and negative. It is positive, since the right is a right of access to the services at the counter. It is arguable whether Smith has a positive right to a post office as such, but certainly Smith has a right of access to this post office's services because it is open to all and is operated at public expense for a public purpose. But Smith's right is also negative, since it is a right against others' interfering with the proper order of her access. And if Smith had to summon the postmaster, a police officer, or the courts to help enforce this negative right, she would be relying on a positive right of access to the protection of public authorities, which, of course, does cost.

One additional element of rights can be elicited from this example. If it is true that all rights rely on some rule, which is itself a part of a social role or institution, what would be the relevant rule and role in the post-office line? If Smith's right to treatment in accordance with her place in line were challenged by Jones, what might Smith say in defense? "These are the rules here, Jones," comes readily to mind. But this is clearly an unhelpful response, since it amounts to a mere restatement of the rule and is not the justification of the rule that is being demanded. A better response to the challenge might be that serving customers in turn reflects a commitment to the "first come, first served" rule and that such a rule creates an orderly system of service. The moral importance of order lies in the other social goods it creates: efficiency, regularity, dependabilty, and the like. But all these virtues of order could be had by other rules as well. A rule of the shortest (or tallest) first would create order. So would a rule of the strongest or smartest first. (Imagine a small testing area near the counter.) The post office could both raise revenue and spread its crowds across the whole day by allowing open bidding: those willing to pay the most go first. There could be a two-tiered postal system: one with first-class service for those able and willing to pay for it, and one with minimal service for those who cannot or choose not to pay. There might be a rule that those who use the postal system most (or least) always go first. We might allow those who contribute most to society to go to the head of the line. (Special passes could be issued.) We could even use race and gender to form separate lines. There are probably endless ways to generate order and the efficiency, regularity, and dependability it generates.

These fanciful possibilities suggest that it is not simply the value of the order derived from the rule of first come, first served that generates a right to go in turn. Although order is certainly a value here, it can be achieved in other ways that we would reject as absurd or invidious. Instead, the main moral value preserved by the post-office rule is the social role it ascribes to persons. It creates equal moral standing for each person at the post office. Regardless of strength, social contribution, money, race, and other determinants, each individual is accorded a certain respect, a certain role as a person with equal moral dignity, when access is determined only by virtue by his or her place in line. This indicates that one very important aspect of rights is the respect for individuals that they establish.[6] Another person should not be served ahead of Smith on the post-office line simply because Smith has the same moral standing as everyone else there. As Smith waited her turn, so should Jones and all the others. Any other rule (used on a routine basis) would probably be a violation of the most basic moral right: the right to be accorded a role as a person equal in moral standing to other persons. This point illuminates the earlier observation that entitlement itself and not the substance of what one is entitled to sometimes creates the seriousness of a rights claim. If entitlement secures the equal moral standing of persons, then entitlement is itself a morally serious concern, regardless of the specifics of the claim at hand.

Finally, rights have an important relationship to justice. Treating persons the way they are morally entitled to be treated is the heart of justice. More may be required by other moral virtues, as the case of Jones's infant suggests, but justice in social relationships demands the creation of guarantees so that persons are treated as they are entitled to be. Put negatively, a society that routinely violates the rights of persons cannot be considered just, whatever else it may or may not be. A post office where the strong always stepped ahead of the weak, for example, would be an unjust social institution because the rights of the weak were being violated. Therefore, determining the rights of persons and the justice of a society are closely related enterprises.

In sum, the important features of rights include these. Rights are serious entitlements derived from social rules and institutional roles. These rules and roles may be the more or less explicit ones of law or the vaguer ones of morality. Rights are socially guaranteed by virtue of the duties they entail for others. They are relinquishable by their possessors and sometimes for good moral reasons. Although usually binding, they may sometimes be overridden by other rights or by extreme circumstances. Rights may be negative protections from interference, positive means of access, or both. Rights have an important relationship to respect for the equal moral dignity of persons. Finally, respect for persons' rights is tied directly to the determination of the justice of a society.

If it makes sense to speak of rights in the relatively insignificant context of a post-office line, does it make sense to speak of rights in the far more important context of health care? Is there a right to health care? The main purpose of the rest of this chapter is to explore the theoretical bases on which this question can be answered. It will be useful to begin with a brief overview of some of the major reasons for and against an affirmative answer.

For and against a right to health care

There is an evident sense in which there are rights within health care in the relatively insignificant sense in which there is a right to be served in turn in a post office. If the first come, first served rule prevails in a doctor's office, a clinic, or another health care setting, a right similar to that in the post-office line may exist. But this is not the interesting and significant sense of right in which some have claimed a right to health care. Rather, the relevant sense of this right is a right of access to the personnel and institutions that care for and sometimes cure those with health care needs.

If the question of the existence of a right to health care is interpreted legally, the answer in general in the United States is negative. A right to health care is not guaranteed in the Constitution, nor does it appear to follow legally from any of the substantive rights set out in that document.[7]

Of course, the federal and state governments have established certain categorical and needs-based programs, Medicare and Medicaid in particular, and those qualifying for these programs may be said to have legal rights to the benefits they convey. There are also laws and regulations that forbid the denial of health care on discriminatory grounds and that mandate that certain levels of care be given to certain categories of needy individuals— handicapped newborns, for example.[8] And a growing trend in the American law of torts may amount to a virtual guarantee of needed emergency care at a hospital emergency room under some circumstances.[9] From an even wider legal perspective, the United States has signed the United Nations Universal Declaration of Human Rights, which calls for universal recognition of a right to health care.[10] Indeed, such a right is recognized to one degree or other in every industrialized democracy except the United States and the Republic of South Africa.[11] In spite of these qualifications, the answer to the legal question is no: there is no general legal right to health care in the United States.

But the real point of the question of a right to health care, its reformist edge, is the moral issue that it raises. Is there a moral right to health care, or, more appropriately, should we recognize a moral right to health care? What moral rules or institutional roles might provide a basis for such a moral entitlement? Of course, the moral issue cannot be held completely separate from the legal issue. If there is a persuasive basis for a moral right to health care, it might then be incumbent on a just society to effect that moral right by institutionalizing a corresponding legal right. In other words, if reasonable and morally sensitive people ought to acknowledge a right to health care, then a just society is probably bound to guarantee that entitlement with the force of law. But must reasonable and morally sensitive people acknowledge a moral right to health care?

One attempt to provide a basis for a claim of a moral right to health care might begin by pointing to the good consequences that would likely follow from the recognition of such a right, and the bad consequences that would likely be avoided.[12] It seems plausible to assume that one of the very basic moral rules is a general obligation to seek to increase the amount of good and decrease the amount of bad in human experience. Surely pain, suffering, disability, and premature death are bad states to be avoided when possible. Health care is frequently effective in palliating pain and suffering and in preventing disability and premature death. It has already been shown, for example, that in many nations where basic health care is considered to be a matter of right, the infant mortality rate is lower and life expectancy is longer than in the United States.[13] And some of the relative successes of the limited right to health care secured for some Americans by Medicare and Medicaid have also been documented in Chapter 1. Thus health care appears to be a powerful instrumental good, a social means of bringing about good consequences and avoiding bad. If acknowledgment of a right to health care would tend to increase access to appropriate health care, more good would then be created as a consequence and more bad would be avoided. More pleasures would replace pains; there would be more happiness and less suffering; and more people would lead longer, more complete lives.

In addition to the direct increase in good and decrease in bad experiences for individuals that the recognition of a right to health care might generate, there might be indirect social goods. Guaranteed access to health care might provide an incentive, or at least remove a disincentive, to seek preventive care before illness strikes and to seek treatment earlier when it does. This might well lower costs overall. With less illness and a more generally healthy population, work productivity and the general quality of life would likely be enhanced. A healthier population is a national asset in innumerable ways. So too is the sense of civic fellowship and social solidarity that the guarantee of entitlement to health care might tend to generate.[14] Thus one approach to grounding a moral right to health care is by reference to the morally significant consequences that might follow from it. Broadly, this approach is utilitarian because it underscores the moral usefulness of guaranteeing universal entitlement to health care.

Drawing on the earlier observation that one fundamental function of rights is to establish roles that provide equal respect for persons, an entirely different approach suggests itself. An argument for a moral right to health care can be made on egalitarian grounds without appealing to consequences.[15] As persons, we are all equally subject to pain, suffering, disability, and death. The need for health care is universal and largely unpredictable. Although many diseases and causes of death are related to personal choices for which individuals may bear some degree of responsibility, many more are plainly not related to choice and more again are ambiguously related to choice. Being born with a genetic defect or a genetic disposition for a disease is beyond a person's conscious choice. So too is all aging and most dying. There may be some assignable responsibility for injuries sustained in a traffic accident, but certainly not to all those who are injured. Even in the cases of diseases related to life style, it is difficult in any given case to determine the extent of personal responsibility in light of the multitude of genetic and cultural factors at work. Our diseases and death may vary in particular, but each of us is equally subject to them in general regardless of our choices. Respect for the equal dignity of persons therefore entails a commitment to equal access to the means necessary to cope with these burdens. Furthermore, our system of providing health care is made possible only because of substantial public investment in health-sciences education, hospital construction, medical research, regulation of the quality of care and its payment, and so on.[16] It seems fitting in light of these public investments that the public have access to the fruits of that investment in some broadly equal fashion. Finally, recognition of a moral right to health care would also be consistent with the divine grounding of equal human dignity proclaimed by our major religious traditions.[17] If all persons stand equal before God, then perhaps they ought to have equal access to such a needed basic service as health care.

A third approach to establishing the grounds for a right to health care is based on consideration of the obligations that arise from membership in a politically organized society.[18] One way to conceptualize these obligations is to think of them as following from an implicit contract among all members of a society. If the implicit social contract that morally binds citizens in a political society includes the duty to ensure that all the members of that society have access to some level of health care, then those individuals have a moral right to that level of care. Since no social contract is available for inspection as a matter of fact, speculation is required to determine what reasonable persons would agree to, if they were placed in the position of having to determine the most basic rules of fairness in society. To ensure their own impartiality, the contractors can be imagined to be behind a "veil of ignorance," which denies them knowledge about their own factual standing in the society for which they are composing rules. Thus, for example, they would be unaware of their own race, gender, social and financial positions, and health care needs. Under these hypothetical conditions, it is plausible to assume that reasonable contractors would agree to rules that give each of them the best prospects for life in the real society regardless of what actual individual situations turn out to be. Since none of the contractors knows his or her own health status and needs, it seems plausible to think that they would agree to a guarantee for all citizens of the largest minimum amount of health care consistent with the social system as defined by the other rules to which they agree. But if this is what reasonable and wholly unbiased persons would agree to as fair if they were forging a morally binding social contract, then this is what real persons ought to agree to in real societies if they are to be reasonable, unbiased, and fair. If, from a moral point of view, we ought to guarantee a minimum amount of health care as an entitlement following from an implicit social contract, then we ought to recognize a right to that level of care.

These, then, are three of the main approaches to justifying an affirmative answer to the question, Is there a right to health care? The utilitarian approach focuses on the likely production of good consequences and avoidance of bad consequences that would follow from acting on a right to health care. The egalitarian approach grounds the claim of right on the fundamental moral equality of persons and the respect for that status that a right to health care would establish. The contractarian approach holds that in our present real society, we are morally bound to agree to what would be agreed to by reasonable, unbiased, and fair persons and that such persons would agree to recognize a right to health care. There are, of course, rejoinders to each of these claims. It can be argued, for example, that in terms of consequences, more bad than good would likely issue from a right to health care. The notion of respect for the dignity of persons might be rejected or its egalitarian implications for health care denied. The social-contract approach might be dismissed as too hypothetical, or it might be argued that reasonable contractors would not agree to a right to health care.

More important than these rejoinders, however, is an alternative understanding of the nature of rights that restricts the application of rights to negative rights only.[19] For libertarians, the fundamental rights are liberty rights of noninterference. On this account, persons have inherent rights to life, liberty, and property. Political society's only function is to see that these basic rights are not violated and to provide just compensation when they are. Any social contract is thus limited to an obligation to create the police and judicial powers needed to enforce these rights and to rectify violations of them. People are free to acquire and exploit the resources of nature and to exchange these resources and the goods and services based on them among themselves. What is just in a libertarian society is any result that is the product of individuals' just original acquisitions and their subsequent choices to buy, sell, freely give, or otherwise transfer resources justly. The so-called positive rights of access are unjustified demands against someone else's liberty or property. But there can be no straightforward positive right to another's liberty or property. Specifically, there can be no right to health care because it would entail an unjustified demand for health care goods and services not owned by the claimant. Thus it would violate the liberty and property rights of health care personnel and owners of health care resources.[20] The libertarian position need not be callous to the plight of those without the private means to secure access to health care. Personal charity, voluntary organizations' assistance, and even government efforts to provide or finance health care are compatible with some versions of libertarianism. There is even the possibility that some amount and kinds of charity in health care contexts is morally obligatory.[21] What is essential to the libertarian perspective, however, is the denial that people are entitled to health care. For libertarians, there can be no right to what is not personally owned. Strictly speaking, the only primary right to health care would be held by those who possess the skills and resources to provide it.

If it could be shown that the present possession of health care skills and resources resulted from injustices in their original acquisition or in the history of their subsequent transfers to contemporary persons and institutions, a different result would follow. Then it would be incumbent on government to rectify these past injustices. If the individuals and the heirs of the individuals who were treated unjustly in this process could not be identified, a systemic compensation might be appropriate. This could take the form of recognition of a right to health care for all, since such an entitlement would ensure that all those wronged receive access to the care they might otherwise have secured for themselves. Hence, even libertarianism can provide a basis for a right to health care, a compensatory right designed to rectify past injustices.

These four views on the right to health care—utilitarianism, egalitarianism, contractarianism, and libertarianism—will be examined in more detail in the chapters that follow. Two important issues must be kept on the horizon of this examination, one of which has already been touched on. If a right to health care is a guarantee of entitlement, access to care cannot be based simply on the ability to pay—unless it were the case, as it clearly is not, that everyone entitled to care is also able to pay for it. The ability to pay may be made part of a scheme to guarantee access to the care that a right to health care would entail, but it cannot be the sole criterion. If there is a right to health care, it is an entitlement to care regardless of the ability to pay. The second issue is suggested by the first. If a right to health care is a guarantee of access to care, all or part of which entitled individuals cannot pay for, then someone else must bear these costs. The dimensions of the costs involved have been outlined in Chapter 1. They are already immense and potentially limitless. Thus the second point: any reasonable claim for a right to health care must have limits.

3
Utilitarianism

Optimal consequences

A first approximation of a theory of persons' rights to health care in a just society can be supplied by exploring utilitarian moral theory.[1] This theory is inspired by an empirical disposition that seeks to locate the rightness or wrongness of an act by reference to the tendency of the act to generate good or bad consequences. It is thus outcome oriented. The moral act is that act whose consequences have the greatest moral utility. This act tends to realize the greatest possible amount of good, the least possible amount of bad, or the best possible ratio of good to bad. Utilitarianism thus insists on measuring the morality of an act by the empirical upshot of the act and not by any theoretical claims about the rightness or wrongness of the nature of the act in and of itself. So, for example, a utilitarian would not judge lying to be somehow wrong by its nature. Instead, a utilitarian would probably judge lying to be wrong by virtue of the bad consequences usually generated by lies: the alienation of those lied to, the manipulative traits engendered in the liar, and the breakdown in social trust. Lying is wrong because it produces these moral disutilities.

Immediately apparent is one of the strengths of utilitarianism. It draws attention to the point, or certainly one of the points, of morality—the difference that it makes empirically in the lives of persons. Lies generally hurt someone, and it is the palpably bad experience of hurting that makes lying wrong. Acts judged right are typically neutral in consequence, or they produce some kind of positive moral utility: human pleasure, happiness, or other sorts of satisfaction. In a concrete situation of moral choice, the utilitarian theory provides a clear and readily appreciated focus. How will each possible course of action affect the pleasure or pain, happiness or unhappiness, and satisfaction or frustration of those involved? Likely outcomes having been determined, it is then morally incumbent on the utilitarian to choose the consequentially optimal course of action.

Apparent also is a second strength of utilitarianism: its flexibility. If the empirical consequences of an act differ in differing circumstances, so will its moral character. Not all lies, for example, produce disutilities. Generally, the trivial white lie does not produce negative consequences and therefore is not morally condemned. One can imagine many circumstances in which important lies might actually produce good results or avoid exceptionally bad ones: a lie to protect an innocent person or a whole society from attack, a lie to an enemy in a just war, a lie to hide a damaging truth about a friend, a lie to build confidence or to help another cope with disaster, a lie to help expose worse lies. The point is not that these lies are necessarily good, but that they can be good depending on the circumstances. If we know that such lies can be good, an acceptable moral theory ought to be able to tell us why. Utilitarianism does: when the consequences are good, the act is good.

Because utilitarianism is a genuine moral theory and not merely a calculation of personal advantage, the pleasure, happiness, and satisfaction of all those involved must be counted neutrally and equally. Neutrality requires that moral choice be unbiased, that it avoid the egoism so natural to personal prudence. Utilitarianism does not mandate altruism to the detriment of the ego, but it does mandate, in quite traditional terms, that others be considered as oneself. This imperative is sometimes expressed metaphorically by the notion of a benevolent spectator. One should choose from such a spectator's point of view—that is, as though one had no active stake in the outcome except to see that good consequences are maximized or, when that is impossible, that bad consequences are minimized. And the same number of good or bad consequences for one person must be weighed the same as that for any other.

Calculating and seeking the largest aggregate utility are thus at the heart of the utilitarian project. In real circumstances, such a quantitative approach will rarely be precise. Consider a simple case. Suppose that an employer has a limited amount of resources to distribute as health care benefits to the company's employees. How can one measure precisely the various utilities possible? What are the moral consequences of dividing the money for benefits equally among all the employees, rather than providing better coverage to just a few, perhaps to those with greater health care needs or to the more senior employees? Yet even though precision in calculation is not possible, something very much like calculation does occur when possible outcomes are projected. Equal, minimally adequate benefits for all, for example, will probably make everyone happy, but only marginally. All benefits for just a few makes those few happy, but not the others. If some employees need the benefits more or deserve them more, perhaps the others will understand; but perhaps not. And possible complaints and poor morale are surely to be counted as disutilities. No doubt, many considerations of just this sort are involved in any serious choice affecting others. So while the precision suggested by the concepts of calculation and maximization of utility is not mathematical, something very much like a "sizing up" or a "weighing of alternatives" is certainly a large and crucial part of moral deliberation and choice.

The quantitative dimension of utilitarianism becomes more evident when the focus of the calculation is changed. In the case of distributing health care benefits, it was implied that the utility of a situation is to be judged only by reference to that single situation, to that single act of distribution. This application of the theory is act utilitarianism, by which the principle of utility is applied directly to single acts and their individual consequences. But utilitarianism can also be applied only indirectly to single acts and directly to rules and policies. This is rule utilitarianism, by which the principle of utility is applied to a rule or system of rules and policies. Under rule utilitarianism, single acts are morally justified by the utility of the rule or policy that governs them, whether or not the acts themselves maximize utility in their own specific circumstances. For example, suppose there is a significant turnover of employees and changing pressures in the health insurance environment, so that the choice of a company's package of health care benefits is not a once-and-for-all choice, but an ongoing one. In that case, a rule for distribution over a number of individual acts of distribution is needed. Other things being equal, perhaps providing the same benefits to all employees has the most overall utility. But other methods have to be considered, especially when other things are not equal. There may be fundamental disagreement about the nature of health care benefits. Are health care benefits deserved in any sense? Should they be regarded as a right, or can they be conceived as incentives or rewards? What if some employees want expanded maternity coverage but others want protection against the costs of nursing-home care? Suppose some employees want to forgo any health care benefits for their equivalent cash value? All these kinds of considerations enter into a determination of the optimal rule for distribution. Whatever rule is ultimately selected based on its overall utility, the benefits can then be distributed according to the rule irrespective of particular daily utilities. Even if today's distribution is not morally optimal, the rule is an assurance that behavior in conformity with it will produce an optimal result in the long run.

Rule utilitarianism has two important features that are worth considering. First, unlike act utilitarianism, rule utilitarianism provides a meaningful way to speak of persons' rights. For act utilitarianism, whether an employee has a "right" to health care benefits will depend on the calculus of utilities at hand—that is, on whether giving benefits to this person maximizes utility in this situation. But if having a right means being entitled to have something, then act utilitarianism really has no concept of a right. Put another way, having a right to health care benefits means that a person is entitled to them whether or not it maximizes utility for that person to have them. A right could almost be defined as that which is due to a person regardless of the balance of utilities at hand, an entitlement not to be overruled by considerations of utility. So a simple act utilitarianism cannot produce rights. Rule utilitarianism, on the contrary, can allow for a derivative concept of a right. An employee's right to health care benefits may be based on the utility produced by the rule for the distribution of benefits, and the rule determines that today this employee is entitled to receive these benefits. A rule-utilitarian right, then, is derived from the overall utility secured by a rule or policy that guarantees certain entitlements to persons. The connection of rights with justice is made clear here, too. Under an act-utilitarian scheme, one could never say that the health care benefits in a company were distributed unjustly, only that better consequences could have been attained by a different distribution. Under rule utilitarianism, one can say that the distribution is unjust if the justifying rule is not followed. If it is not followed, it is likely that someone's rights are being violated. This is prima facie unjust.

The second important feature of rule utilitarianism is that it provides a moral framework for policy choice. Quantification is usually a prominent element, and questions concerning the social implications of the policy are generated. What impact does a proposed policy have on persons' pleasure, happiness, and satisfaction in general? How many people are affected, and for how long? What are the financial and other social costs of various policy alternatives? How efficient a use of inevitably scarce resources is this choice, compared with other choices? Which other opportunities are lost and which are created by choosing this option? Does the proposed policy have an impact on other rules and policies? Will new rights be generated and old ones compromised or enhanced? The virtue of rule utilitarianism lies not only in raising these questions as explicitly moral issues, but also in doing so outside the context of individual choice. The pressures of personality and circumstance may cloud clear moral thinking in the distribution of a package of health care benefits to an individual employee, but in the detachment characteristic of an ideal policy choice, all factors can be properly considered and each given its due weight. Furthermore, rule utilitarianism applied to policy choices can easily average the good and bad consequences over the number of persons affected by the policy. Whereas classical act utilitarianism seeks simply the largest net aggregate of good over bad, average rule utilitarianism can choose on the basis of the average difference that a policy makes in the long run. This avoids certain classical problems having to do with measuring the effects of extremely good or bad consequences for a small number of persons and with accounting for changes in the total number of persons affected by a choice. Average rule utilitarianism provides moral grounds for adopting policies that optimize the average consequences for all those the policies affect.

In spite of the benefits of average rule utilitarianism, certain theoretical problems remain for utilitarianism. These problems are important to recognize, since they have a bearing on the application of utilitarianism to the question of a right to health care. Three difficulties stand out.

First, the problem of the imprecision of calculation remains for utilitarianism, even when the focus is on rules and policies. In the simple case of employee health care benefits, for example, what weight should be given to the utility of equal treatment over time compared with the utility that might be gained by using health care benefits as an incentive? Under the former policy, the employees receive equal protection (assuming equal need for the benefits), and satisfaction is secured and disappointment avoided by everyone's having equal standing over time. But suppose the employees' productivity could be improved in ways that would profit them in the long run by using the health care benefits as an incentive. If individual benefits were tied to individual productivity, for example, the profitability of the entire company might be raised to the point that a larger total package of health benefits could be made available for distribution or more money might be available for salary increases. Allowance could even be made for effort or improvement, so that some benefits could sometimes go to the employees with the overall worst productivity if they seemed to be trying harder. Is it not possible that the net happiness produced by this policy could be larger than that attained by the equal-benefits policy on average and in the long run? How could one be sure? How could one measure the utility of the security produced by the policy of equal distribution versus the utility of the risk and excitement built into the policy of incentives? Although there still may be a "rough-and-ready" sense in which one can intuitively judge these matters, such intuitions are a long way from the empirical promise of utilitarianism, even at the rule level.

Second, because act utilitarianism can have no coherent concept of rights, it has an obvious problem with justice. It is theoretically incapable of judging a situation to be just or unjust because it attends to only the aggregate outcome. Only the end can justify the means. Rule utilitarianism improves on this shortcoming by allowing for the derivation of rights from rules. But precisely because the rights are derivative, rule utilitarianism may have its own problem with justice. Can a rule be such that overall and on average it maximizes utilty but is at the same time unjust to some of the persons it affects? Strictly speaking, if justice is directly connected with rights and rights are defined only by reference to utility-maximizing rules, then the answer must be no. Theoretically, it cannot be unjust to be treated according to the rules that define rights and therefore justice. But this does not seem adequate to the common-sense, intuitive meaning of justice. Suppose, for example, that three-quarters of the company's employees are exceptionally bright, readily motivated by incentives, and generally in good health. Improving their productivity will likely yield many positive utilities for themselves and for others for a long time to come. The other quarter, let us suppose, are low in intelligence, impervious to incentives, and on the whole in poorer states of health than their other co-workers. Suppose that all the variables involved could be calculated, and the result indicated that an incentive policy for the distribution of employee health care benefits maximized average utility overall. Might we not still be inclined to say that the incentive policy, even admitting its overall utility, is unjust to the last quarter of the employees? Might we not be inclined to say that in some sense, the rights of these employees are violated by a policy that will distribute benefits so disproportionately to others? And even if the incentive policy maximizes utility on average and in the long run, would it not be legitimate for these employees to insist that their needs are not average and their lives are not lived in the long run. Thus rights derivative from rules seem not to suffice, if the rule itself generates a result that seems unjust. If a rule can maximize utility and still be considered unjust, then rule utilitarianism itself has a problem with justice.

The third problem is the relative instability of the distinction between act and rule utilitarianism. The very strengths of the utilitarianism approach are its empirical character and its flexibility. But commitment to rule utilitarianism, while it creates a more stable moral theory in general, sacrifices these virtues to a great extent. Any given rule or policy that is good overall may dictate many individual acts whose empirical consequences in particular circumstances are bad on balance. Adherence to a policy of distributing health care benefits as an incentive or a policy of condemning lies may work in general, but may have just the wrong results in specific circumstances for specific persons today. Rules justify themselves on average and in the long run, but people live their lives as individuals and in the short run. The moral psychology that makes the empirical relevance of utilitarianism attractive in general, makes rule utilitarianism hard to maintain in some contexts. And inflexibility in the application of the rule in particular cases, which is required to maintain rule utilitarianism, runs counter to the other strength of the theory in general—its flexibility in judging good that which brings about good and bad that which brings about bad. But if in fact there is a temptation for the rule utilitarian to slip into act utilitarianism, the already attenuated concept of rights available to the rule utiltarian will be further jeopardized, since act utilitarianism can have no concept of rights.

These are important difficulties, ones not to be ignored in either the theory or the application of utilitarian moral thinking. Yet this theory remains one of the most persuasive options available for a comprehensive moral theory. It indicates where to look: empirical consequences. It says why: they matter for people. It prescribes how to choose: maximize good, minimize bad. And it is, more with act and less with rule, flexible in changing circumstances.

Prudent insurance

In the health care context, the distinction between act and rule utilitarianism presents itself as that between questions of microallocation and of macroallocation, respectively.[2] Microallocation is the moral question of how much care a particular patient should receive in a particular set of circumstances. Cast in utilitarian terms, the microallocation question involves a determination of the care that is cost-beneficial for this patient, sizing up the good and bad consequences at stake for this individual alone. The question may sometimes be comparative, such as the amount of time a nurse should spend with one patient, given the needs and demands of other patients. Either way, the mark of the microallocation question is its contextual character, its direct relevance to an action in a given set of circumstances.

The macroallocation question pertains to the making of policy choices. Utilitarian considerations can be focused in two ways. First, how much of our collective resources should go into health care compared with other social needs? Second, how should those resources be distributed within the health care arena? Both these kinds of choices are to be made on the grounds of expected utility, on average and in the long run. These macroallocation decisions will generate certain derivative rights, usually legal as well as moral rights. Consider, for example, the logic of the moral reasoning behind the establishment of the series of policy choices institutionalized in the Medicare program. Amid all the political considerations at its inception, there were also the moral concerns of the utility to be expected from these policy choices compared with the utility to be gained by other choices or none at all. Analytically, two levels of rule-utilitarian judgments can be distinguished in the establishment of the program. (This is not a claim about how the program was established in fact, but about the moral logic of its establishment.) First, a judgment had to be made about the relative benefits of money spent on health care rather than on, say, education or defense.

Second, a judgment had to be made about the relative benefits of a health care program for those over age sixty-five and with certain disabilities rather than, say, a health care program for pregnant women or for the unemployed. Once these choices were made and the program was established, those covered by the program gained derivative moral and legal rights to the benefits made available. The projected utilities that justified the program generated the rights.

But the key moral question at stake is whether a right to health care of some broad (although inevitably limited) character should be recognized. The answer to such a question cannot be based solely on rights generated under existing programs, but must rest on the balance of utilities that might be achieved under possible policies. Rule utilitarianism mandates the choice of the consequentially optimal social rules, and its derivative moral rights follow from those projected consequences. Therefore, if there is a rule-utilitarian case to be made for a moral right to health care, it must follow from the projected utilities of a policy that guarantees entitlement to some degree of health care.

Obviously, the first place to turn for an estimate of projected utilities from a right to health care are the human needs on which health care is predicated.[3] Illness and disability are potent sources of physical pain for those who suffer from them, and one time or another, all of us do. Illness and disability can also bring unhappiness and frustration of other possible satisfactions both for the sufferer and for those who love, depend on, or care for the sufferer. Premature death is not empirically a direct pain or unhappiness for the dead, but it can be conceived to be the ultimate frustration of other possible satisfactions, especially the basic satisfaction of having empirical experience itself. It probably is this loss of opportunity for the satisfactions of any sort of empirical experience that accounts for the universal evaluation of early and preventable death as a tragedy for the deceased. There is also considerable pain, unhappiness, and frustration suffered by those who loved, befriended, or even just knew the victim of premature death. Simply stated, and substantially understated, pain, suffering, and frustration are the disutilities widely created by illness, disability, and premature death.

For most of its long history, health care could do little to prevent or minimize such disutilities.[4] When health care could make little empirical difference, the position that there is a right of access to it could have little utilitarian support. But the flexibility of utilitarian moral reasoning is apparent. Now that a medical armamentarium of great efficacy exists, a much more powerful rule-utilitarian argument for access to it can be made. To simplify the point considerably, suppose that a community has an ongoing rate of physical pain measured (presuming for the moment that it can be measured precisely) at 1,000 disutilities annually. If the best health care effort possible costs the community 300 utilities in financial support (which could have gone elsewhere) and the amount of pain is lowered by, say, only 100 disutilities, then the ratio of good to bad consequences is such that no plausible case for a derivative right to health care can be mounted. But suppose that the same investment in the same community two generations later could lower the amount of pain by 600 disutilities. These consequences would be such that a policy guaranteeing access to health care might be justified. In that case, a prima facie case for a derivative right to health care could be made. Pretense of precision aside, the power of contemporary health care puts us closer to the later community than to the earlier. Humans have a basic need to avoid pain, suffering, and frustration, and health care can now satisfy that need in many cases. If the moral utilities are anywhere near those of the later community, then we ought to satisfy that need by adopting a social policy of guaranteeing access to health care. Adoption of such a policy would entail a derivative right to health care.

Consider this rejoinder, however. Admitting the efficacy of contemporary health care and the basic nature of the need for it, it still may not follow that maximum utility lies in the direction of employing social resources to serve that need. To use social resources entails not only a direct financial cost, but also the associated costs of increased government bureaucracy (someone will have to guarantee the right) and taxation of private individuals and activities (the source of social resources). Furthermore, other basic needs, such as food, clothing, and shelter, are not guaranteed by right and supported by social resources. Does it not create more utility in light of these considerations to let individuals use private resources to buy and sell health care services in a free market, just as we allow for the commercial distribution of food, clothing, and shelter?

Three utilitarian responses can be made to this rejoinder. First, it may well be that analogous rule-utilitarian arguments can be made for a moral responsibility to guarantee a right to food, clothing, and shelter, sufficient at least to cover persons' basic needs.[5] Not everyone is able to buy enough of these necessities or of basic health care because of the general inequity in persons' economic circumstances. In this context, much avoidable pain, suffering, and frustration is generated. Entitlement to satisfaction of all these basic needs would avoid these disutilities and, depending on an assessment of the relevant costs, would likely be justified as a rule. Indeed, one might say that the various human-welfare policies adopted by virtually all industrialized democracies in the twentieth century represent a practical acknowledgment of the force of the argument that can be made in favor of an entitlement to some satisfaction of all basic needs. When social resources are such that with a reasonably favorable ratio of good to bad consequences, they can be used to satisfy basic human needs, then they ought to be. This is merely another way of stating the rule-utilitarian principle. So the first response to the free-market rejoinder is that the analogy to the way food, clothing, and shelter is distributed cuts both ways. Perhaps from the moral point of view, there ought to be a more explicit derivative right to these basics as well as to basic health care.

Second, health care needs may in fact differ from other basic needs in ways that make it more important that health care be distributed as a matter of entitlement and not in a commercial context.[6] The basic needs for food, clothing, and shelter are relatively constant for all persons, and therefore are highly predictable. Although each of us has or will have a need for basic health care, some of those needs are highly variable and therefore unpredictable. Who can say, for example, if or when they will be taken unconscious to a hospital emergency room, the victim of someone else's driving error? When the need for health care does occur, when an infant has a high and unresponsive fever, for example, the need is pressing, urgent. Few economic trade-offs are appropriate; shopping for bargains and waiting for sales are out of the question.

In the context of care itself—say, having a suspicious lump examined—treatment options are nonstandard. By contrast, nearly any food will do when one is hungry; when cold, nearly any clothes and shelter. Because of the scientific and clinical experience needed to determine proper health care, patients and potential patients must rely on health care professionals' expertise. Patients are often incapable of judging the quality of the health care they have received. Sometimes the very best care will still have the worst outcome. Because of the body's natural ability to heal and the mind's clear role in the placebo effect, patients are often unable to even appraise the efficacy of their care even when they regain health. Compared with consumers of food, clothing, and shelter, patients are thus in an exceptionally dependent relationship with providers. Because of the reliance and vulnerability that this dependence creates for the patient, the satisfaction of health care needs requires a degree of trust far beyond anything necessary for the satisfaction of other basic needs. In health care, therefore, the principle of commerce—"Let the buyer beware"—does not have its usual utility. Hence, even if it could be shown that the needs for food, clothing, and shelter were best satisfied not by a rule creating an entitlement, but by free exchange in the marketplace, it would not follow that health care was similarly best distributed. The need for health care differs from other basic needs in ways that may mandate the adoption of rules establishing a right to it.

Finally to the rejoinder, it must be admitted that financial and other social costs must be weighed in considering utilitarian grounds for a right to health care. The amount of money invested in health care will have to be justified by reference to projected results. The taxation of private individuals and activities is a social cost, especially if its effect is to dampen the creation of wealth in society in general. This is a moral concern, since a general reduction of wealth reduces correspondingly the amount of resources in principle available to satisfy basic needs and thus raises the price of satisfying them. An impoverished society, for an extreme example, may have so many other unmet needs and so few resources that the cost of satisfying basic health care needs rises to the point that rule utilitarianism could not justify considering health care to be a derivative right. Short of this sort of damaging economic effect of overtaxation or general impoverishment, rule-utilitarian theory can have no in principle objection to taxation for any public purpose that justifies itself in long-term consequences. It seems reasonable to assume that although the cost of health care is high and continues to rise, American society is not at the stage where health care–related taxation is eroding the wealth necessary to afford the provision of such care as an entitlement, given appropriate limits. Certainly, the general affluence of American life is prima facie evidence in support of this assumption.

There is a social cost of sorts associated with the growth of government and government bureaucracy.[7] For any number of reasons, not the least of which is the social utility of a healthy degree of individuality, it would be best if the entitlement to health care could be guaranteed in ways that minimized this growth. But the same rule applies elsewhere as well. Wherever the government must act, the least necessary is to be preferred. Yet if the balance of all the other consequences of entitling citizens to some degree of health care is favorable, the negative character of the growth of government would have to be especially strong to overrule recognition of a moral right to health care. As long as our traditions of democratic, citizen control over government and of individual initiative remain strong, the fear of growth of government will not be persuasive enough to overrule the utilty of preventing much pain, suffering, disability, and premature death by guaranteeing a right to health care. Furthermore, there is a positive side to a bureaucratic response to a social need that ought not to be overlooked.[8] Public investment in an institution designed to satisfy persons' basic needs can be a potent rallying point for social ideals of solidarity and civic fellowship. For example, in Great Britain, the place of origin of many of our democratic and individualist traditions, the National Health Service is second only to the Crown in institutional popularity.[9]

If it is insufficient on grounds of utility to leave the distribution of health care largely to the marketplace—and certainly, the empirical failings of the American system of distribution suggest this—what amount of our social resources is appropriately spent on health care, and where is it best spent? Obviously, the context of an account of the moral grounds for the basis of a claim to a right to health care is not the place to attempt to answer these questions in terms of dollars and cents. Many practical matters beyond the reach of this investigation have to be considered in determining the proper dimensions of a national health care budget, and this is a matter for ongoing debate and reassessment as empirical realities change. Instead, a reasonable expectation from the perspective of utilitarian moral theory is a verbal formula that can give sense and direction to concrete budgetary discussions.

A useful starting point for devising such a formula can be gained by examining the implications of the so-called law of marginal utility.[10] According to this doctrine, utilitarian reasoning will have a decided bent in the direction of egalitarian distribution schemes because a small amount of resources channeled to those who have little will create more utility than the same amount of resources channeled to those who already have a great deal. Put simply, a dollar is of more consequence to a poor person than to a rich person. The more reduced the circumstances, the more important the dollar; and because the poor person's dollar can be presumed in general to go to satisfy basic needs, the greater the utility. But rule utilitarianism mandates the greatest utility in social policy. Therefore, other things being equal, rule utilitarianism will be disposed toward the distribution of resources that create equal satisfaction of basic needs, including equal access to health care services for basic health care needs.

Utilitarian theory might go further to mandate equalization of all health care, basic and otherwise, except for three considerations. Beyond the satisfaction of basic health care needs, there can be less confidence in the assumption that a dollar is of more value to the less well-off. Although basic human needs are universal, people surely differ in their desires and capacities for satisfaction of those desires.[11] Basic needs having been satisfied, it may not be the case that a dollar means more to a poor person than to a rich person. While it may often be so, the poor person may be easily contented with simple pleasures, whereas the rich person may be driven to excess. In this case, the logic of marginal utility would be reversed. Were society to commit itself to guaranteeing entitlement to the equal satisfaction of the desires of the rich, it would be subsidizing Faustian insatiability, to the detriment of other more pressing basic needs. The achievement of maximum utility cannot lie in this direction.

The second utilitarian consideration that argues against total equality in access to health care resources has been alluded to before. It seems plain that nonegalitarian incentives, at least in the context of the personal acquisitiveness that drives much of contemporary American capitalism, have the ability to increase the amount of wealth in society. It would plainly work against the attainment of the greatest possible utility to prevent the use of incentives, if they help create the resources that, in turn, allow for more widespread satisfaction of basic needs. So rule utilitarianism's egalitarian disposition will be restricted somewhat by the necessity of creating the resources needed to generate maximum good consequences. Although this may result in differential health care, if the use of such incentives yields a higher average utility than any other option, it would be morally justified. There are also other kinds of health care "wealth," including the results of medical experimentation and other health care innovations. It would be prohibitively expensive for society to fund all these ventures directly, but it is a collective benefit to have this sort of wealth. Therefore, even if promoting health care innovations means that some persons are treated more or better than others in relevantly similar circumstances, it can be justified if the innovations are ultimately made available to satisfy the basic needs of the wider public. If nonegalitarian policies can thus increase the health care "pie" and by doing so enhance the average utility of health care, then their use can be justified in spite of the generally egalitarian thrust of the law of marginal utility.

Finally, a commitment to strictly equal satisfaction of health care needs, even basic needs, cannot maximize utility because, depending on the meaning of "basic," the basic needs of some will be too expensive for any society to afford. If basic needs are founded in our natural avoidance of pain, suffering, and frustration, especially including that of premature death, some needs will be such that only a prohibitively expensive investment of social resources will satisfy them. Suppose, for an extreme example, that the only way to avoid the premature death of one person would require the investment of the nation's entire annual health-care budget. Without raising the thorny question of the precise monetary value of saving a life,[12] surely this cost would be too high. The moral point is obvious: everything invested in one person means nothing for anyone else. An average rule utilitarianism could never tolerate this sort of imbalance, even if the stakes for the individual are life and death. This example is extreme, of course, but it serves to establish the principle that rule utilitarianism's general bias toward equal satisfaction of basic health care needs must have limits.

What all of this means is that the moral imperative of rule utilitarianism would probably lead us to establish policies that guaranteed entitlement to some reasonable level of satisfaction of basic human needs for all in a system that allowed for the use of incentives for the satisfaction of desires beyond basic needs and of needs beyond what society can afford to satisfy. In terms of health care, this would entail a limited right to basic health care, with the ability to satisfy additional health care desires and uncovered needs in a free market. In other words, rule utilitarianism would likely justify a right to a decent minimum of health care, where decent minimum means satisfaction of basic human health care needs within reasonable limits.[13]

But this formula still needs further development. What is a decent minimum, and what are basic needs? The first is obviously a dynamic notion that must be redefined as society and its health care potential and resources change.[14] The second has a universal core built around the empirical realities of pain, suffering, disability, and premature death, but it is also dynamic because of the health care interventions that have been and will be developed. For example, is a liver transplant costing $250,000, but necessary to prevent premature death, basic health care?[15] Is it part of the services that society should guarantee by way of a decent minimum of health care? Again, there are no definite answers to these questions from the point of view of an ethical theory, but a direction from which these questions should be approached can be offered.[16]

Recall that as a moral theory, utilitarianism binds us to consider others as we would consider ourselves, to judge impartially from the point of view of a benevolent spectator. A hypothetical circumstance may help to clarify this. Suppose that a reasonably prudent person has an overall income that is at a decent minimum—say, 50 percent above a realistic conception of poverty in his or her society. Now suppose that this person must buy private insurance from this income to cover the cost of any health care needs that might arise. To make this person unbiased and universally relevant, place him or her behind a veil of ignorance, thus denying the person knowledge of his or her gender, age, and health status. This person must now decide what kinds of and how much health insurance to buy and must be prepared to pay for the premiums out of his or her decent but minimal income. This person will use utilitarian reasoning because the costs and benefits of various insurance options will have to be weighed against one another, with an eye toward selecting the optimal arrangement of the best coverage at the least sacrifice of disposable income (money reserved to produce other benefits). The reasoning will also be average rule utilitarian because only general knowledge about human health needs will be available, none specific to his or her own case. And reasoning will be relevant to our moral situation, since we must choose for others in the creation of social policy as we would choose for ourselves were we reasonable, prudent, and unbiased—just as this hypothetical person is by definition.

What would such a situated person choose? No doubt, he or she would choose in general the health care insurance that provided the best chances for a long life lived well at even a relatively high cost.[17] This would likely include comprehensive prenatal and pediatric care, since such care would help secure the foundations of such a life. Emergency care for a whole range of likely circumstances would be chosen because of the graphic life-and-death difference that such care can often make. Preventive care that had a statistically good return on investment would be another likely choice.

Primary care would probably be chosen because it would ensure a regular and personal point of entry into the health care system as a whole.[18] Some sort of geriatric care would likely be selected for protection in old age. And some insurance would probably be purchased against being entirely impoverished by catastrophic health care costs. Cost would be a consideration throughout, but the clear benefits of such an insurance package would likely justify the costs involved.

Beyond this point, calculations become more difficult. Protection against specific diseases would be purchased only if the likelihood of contracting the diseases was high, the toll in terms of disutilities was acute, and the costs were reasonable. Insurance for a $250,000 liver transplant would likely not be purchased; a fixed number of covered hospital days might be. Coverage for continuation of care while in a persistent vegetative state would not be bought; coverage for chemotherapy might be. Insurance coverage for prenatal surgery probably would not be included; but coverage for heart disease might be. And one can imagine that these kinds of choices would have to be remade by the hypothetical person as health statistics and costs of care varied and as a decent minimum income tended to purchase more or less in his or her society.

If this thought experiment is instructive, it is because average rule utilitarianism requires that we assume a reasonable, prudent, and unbiased position as we appraise the morally relevant consequences of policy choices. We must choose as this hypothetical person would. The resultant policies will generate a derivative right to health care. In theory, this will mean a right to a decent minimum of health care to cover basic human needs as defined by the kinds and amounts of insurance that would be purchased by a reasonably prudent person behind a veil of ignorance. In practice, this means a rule-utilitarian justification for a right to basic prenatal, pediatric, and primary care; catastrophic coverage, and some levels of preventive and geriatric care.

The three problems with rule utilitarianism cited earlier remain, however. Although the cost–benefit ratio of guaranteeing a right to health care seems positive, there is really no way to afix a quantitative value to pains, sufferings, and frustrations that could have been avoided. How, for example, should a premature death be counted? Thus the best that a rule-utilitarian approach can do with such incalculable values is enumerate the likely costs and benefits involved and then draw an intuitively plausible conclusion.

Second, this account may give rise to problems with justice. Using as a model the hypothetical person who is buying insurance, the basic care that a rule-utilitarian right demands would likely not cover certain very expensive or extremely rare health care needs. This follows because a person behind a veil of ignorance would use costs and average probabilities in selecting insurance coverage. But intuitively, this may be unjust. Someone suffering from a rare disease, for example, might not be entitled to social resources, while someone suffering from a common disease would be. Although such a policy produces the greatest average utility, it appears unjust to the victim of the rare disease.

Finally, it is difficult to maintain the rule component of utilitarianism in practice. Politics and the publicity of special cases of health care needs not covered by a rule-utilitarian calculation place pressures on policy makers to add ad hoc categories of coverage. Moral psychology is such that, justified or not, we are often willing to lavish resources on the rescue of identifiable victims even while ignoring statistically more compelling needs.[19] And rule utilitarianism places exceptional pressures on health care professionals whose historical ethic requires them to place the best interests of their individual patients first. In spite of the good policy argument that can be made on behalf of rule utilitarianism, physicians and nurses will likely find it hard to accept a rule that has strongly negative consequences for a minority or even for one of their patients. But if these pressures should erode commitment to rules, the act-utilitarianism alternative makes any concept of a right to health care untenable.

In spite of these difficulties, rule utilitarianism offers a systematic moral framework for defending a claim for a right to health care. On this account, we are entitled to the health care that would follow from a policy that would maximize good consequences in general. Such a policy would provide the basic health care that a rational and prudent person who earned a decent minimum income would buy insurance to cover.

4

Egalitarianism

One of the problems with utilitarianism, as we have seen, is its implications for justice. Act utilitarianism mandates the consequentially maximum choice in a situation, even if reaching this optimum result appears to work an injustice on one individual or some of the individuals involved. Average rule utilitarianism tempers this tendency by the application of the mandate at the level of rules or policies, thus increasing the likelihood that all interests will be served on average and in the long run of the rule's application to individual cases. But there is still the possibility that a rule that maximizes good consequences on average and in the long run can appear unjust to one or some individuals. The impact of the theory for understanding the concept of a right is analogous to its problem with justice. Act utilitarianism can have no coherent concept of a right. Rule utilitarianism can generate rights, but only derivative rights, which follow from the utility maximized by the rules or policies chosen. These two issues are intertwined. Without the concept of a right, what seems unjust cannot be ruled out in principle. With the concept of only a derivative right, what appears unjust may be a less likely result, but still possible in principle.

It will be helpful to reflect further on this finding. Why is it that moral reasoning without the concept of a right appears to allow injustice? Why is it that the concept of a derivative right still seems insufficiently committed to justice? Consider again the simple case of distributing employee health care benefits. Intuitively, and ignoring consequences, it seems most just to divide the resources allotted for benefits equally among all employees. If the total resources are too few for each employee to receive an adequate package of benefits were they distributed equally, not providing health care benefits to any employees seems fairer than providing them to some employees but not to others. Alternatively put, one can imagine sympathizing with the complaints of those denied benefits under other acts or policies of distribution. One can imagine sympathizing with their claims that their rights have been violated.

It is this intuitive sense of justice and of persons' rights that seems to be omitted in the utilitarian approach. Clearly, judgments about both justice and rights are bound in these cases to a rudimentary moral presumption that persons ought to be treated equally. Even if it does not maximize good consequences to do so, it seems morally proper in itself to share limited resources on an equal basis. Utilitarian approaches by their nature focus moral appraisal on the ends of actions and not on the means taken to arrive at those ends. But the complaint of injustice and violation of right is an assertion that some means of getting to an optimum end may be wrong in themselves. To treat persons unequally, if they are equally situated, seems to be an injustice and a violation of right. These intuitive notions can be given more depth and a firmer theoretical foundation by considering the important notion of person and what that notion entails morally.

Equal intrinsic value

To think of a being as a person is to place that being in a radically different category of value from that generally attached to other beings.[1] A thing, for example, acquires its value relative to other values. It may be considered most beautiful, a work of art, and be highly valued; or it may be common and virtually worthless. It may be personally important, a memento of a special time; yet to others, it has no value. It may be highly useful, the only tool for a job, or merely an object without function. It may fetch a great price in a market economy because it is rare and in demand, or it may have little exchange value. A calculation of a thing's value is always relative to these and to a multitude of other factors. It is thus extrinsic to itself.

By contrast, the value of a person is intrinsic.[2] This value is not dependent on relationships to other values, but is of value in and of itself. Indeed, it is ultimately from the point of view of persons that all other beings come to be valued. People ascribe beauty, personal importance, usefulness, monetary worth, and other values to all beings. If persons did not have an inherent value themselves, it is hard to see how other beings could be so valued. To be the source of values, one must be of value. One might almost say that it is in the very activities characteristic of valuing that persons both display and make their own value.[3] In the richness of the creations of culture, in the strivings of industry and commerce, and in all the achievements that follow from our species' ability to reflect on consciousness itself, persons demonstrate a valuing activity qualitatively unique in nature. When denied this activity and the tacit but categorically positive self-appraisal at its source, humans are reduced personally and culturally. To put the point practically, if a person sincerely believed that he or she were of no value as a person, how long could he or she go on valuing other persons or things, how long could he or she be creative, strive for goals, make earnest commitments? If a whole culture of peole should be made to regard themselves as collectively valueless, is it likely that they could generate any serious public values; is great art, material success, or intellectual accomplishment to be expected of a people denied their own self-worth? In the cases of both individuals and groups, it seems that a tacit sense of being inherently valuable is presupposed and necessary for the cultivation of other personal and social values. In this sense, persons create the value in the world and are thus the world's necessary values.[4]

Since the value of persons comes from within, so to speak, and is not dependent on external relationships, the value of persons is not relative. It does not depend on others' ascription of beauty, usefulness, or price. Hence, it is not to be compared with or ranked against other ascriptions of value. In contrast to the relative price of a thing, for example, a person's value is priceless, incalculable. This point can be made obvious by reflection on the moral wrong of slavery. Humans have accepted slavery as an institution for most of their history as a species because there is a certain logic to it. The weak, individually or collectively, are owned by the strong in exchange for a level of survival. The buying and selling or trading of the enslaved proceeds on the basis of any other commodity exchange: price is determined by the being's beauty, usefulness, or resale value. One can even conceive of an average rule-utilitarian justification for this arrangement. Given a large enough benefit to a large number of nonslaves from a small well-defined group of slaves, the average aggregate of good to bad results might be better with slavery than without it. But the revulsion of the modern moral consciousness to this sort of logic is revealing. Persons are not to be owned like things, not to be bought and sold like commodities. Utility in such a case seems irrelevant. The very notion of having one's value determined in this fashion—that is, relative to external factors—is morally offensive, regardless of consequences. It is a direct indignity to persons.

The uncompromising character of this moral rejection of slavery represents an important moral achievement: recognition of the intrinsic and incalculable value of every individual person. It is not permissible to enslave the weak, the foolish, the socially useless. It is simply not permissible to enslave a person. Thus the moral category of being a person does not depend on any specific empirical attainment, nor is it lost through any specific empirical failing. It follows solely from being a person as such. This standing of being a person with incalculable intrinsic worth may be referred to as the dignity of being a person. The acknowledgment of that fundamental dignity may be termed respect for persons.

Respect for persons based on an acknowledgment of dignity has a direct bearing on the concept of equality. Slavery is the moral abomination that it is because it disrespects persons by valuing them unequally—the master as worthy, the slave as unworthy. All the other negative empirical consequences of slavery follow from the presumption of this unequal moral standing, grounded generally in unequal strength. But from the modern viewpoint, no number of unequal empirical attributes can justify the unequal moral standing presumed by slavery—not unequal strength, intelligence, beauty, wisdom, or other quality. There is, in this view, a fundamental moral equality among persons that precedes all empirical inequalities in importance. Persons must be respected as persons before any special empirical qualities they may have or may lack can be taken into consideration.

The moral demand that persons be respected returns us to the concept of rights. If persons have an incalculable and intrinsic dignity, then there are ways they must be treated and ways they cannot be treated. Slavery is an example of the latter. All of us are duty bound to respect personal dignity and therefore to refrain from enslaving others. From the point of view of others, the duty not to enslave is their right to be free from being enslaved. A general theory of equal human rights can be founded on the duties to respect persons' moral dignity. The key to articulating these rights in theory lies in the contrast between this respect for a person's intrinsic and incalculable value and the calculation of the extrinsic and relative value of a thing. The hallmark of injustice and violation of personal rights is the treatment of a person as though he or she were only of extrinsic and relative value, as though he or she were merely a thing. Generally, this is associated with an arbitrary moral appraisal of one person as more worthy than another. Given the natural disposition of the ego, injustice often has its roots in the placing of one's own projects and interests above the moral standing of other persons, treating them merely as something to be used or ignored rather than as persons to be respected.

This general theory of human rights is egalitarian, since it is based on the claim that as persons we are fundamentally equal. Since we are equal in this fashion, others have a duty to treat us this way and we have a right to be so treated. Rights, then, are basic and equal. Short of being overridden by another right or by a catastrophe that temporarily suspends the normal moral presuppositions of social life, rights are morally prevailing entitlements not to be set aside for reasons of utility.[5] Attempting to enumerate all the moral rights that an egalitarian scheme with this basis would include is not profitable here, and it may not be conceptually possible at this level of abstraction. But this account may be made more concrete by categorizing the rudimentary kinds of rights that respect for persons demands. The articulation of these most basic rights follows from thinking of persons as having three fundamental dimensions and therefore three fundamental interests: the philosophical or moral, the interpersonal or political, and the bodily or medical.[6]

First, if the ultimate basis of all human rights on the egalitarian account is the equal moral standing of all persons, the primary right of each person is to be accorded that standing. Theoretically, this means a right to be respected as an equal and incalculable value. Practically, this means a basic right to be respected by others and, perhaps more important, a basic right to develop a proper sense of self-respect. Broadly, ensuring the right to develop self-respect demands equal rights to protection from assault, to cultural literacy, and to the possibility of forming positive relationships with others without arbitrary barriers. All these rights are lost by the slave but guaranteed in a society that respects persons and sets the conditions for them to respect themselves.[7]

Second, respect for persons entails a right to equality of opportunity. This means equal rights to personal liberty, to the ability to construct and execute a reasonable life plan, and to share in the control of the institutions and policies that shape society and one's own life. These rights create a guarantee of political and interpersonal freedoms.

Finally, respect for persons must include a respect for the necessary empirical conditions of persons, the body and mind—an equal right to be free as far as possible from pain, suffering, disability, and premature death. Practically, this means an equal right to a reasonable share of those basic goods and service known to be necessary for a decent human life, including a right to a job, minimum income support, or provision in kind of the goods necessary for life, as well as a right to a range of social and health care services designed to prevent and minimize psychological and physical suffering, disabilities, and premature death.

There are three major difficulties with an egalitarian framework for rights. The first follows from the fact that in many respects, persons have unequal needs. Given these unequal needs and a commitment to equal treatment, egalitarianism is faced with a dilemma. Either treat people the same way regardless of their unequal needs, thereby using equal procedures and producing unequal results, or treat people in accordance with their unequal needs, thereby using unequal procedures and producing substantively equal results.[8] Suppose, for example, that some of a company's employees prefer expanded maternity coverage and that others prefer a dental plan. Must an egalitarian give all the employees the better maternity coverage or all the dental plan in order to ensure equal treatment? Or must an egalitarian give each employee the plan that he or she prefers so that all are equally satisfied, although unequally treated. What if the alternatives are not so simple? Suppose that producing equal satisfaction among all the employees requires that some of the employees receive considerably more of the company's resources than others; perhaps these employees want comprehensive coverage of long-term custodial care at a cost of 10 or 100 times the cost of enhanced maternity coverage. At what point does this sort of attempt to equalize the result become unfair to the more easily satisfied employees? There is no simple answer to this question because it represents a permanent tension in egalitarianism: procedural equality in treatment versus substantive equality in result.

Another way to make the same important point is this. Egalitarian justice demands that persons in similar situations be treated similarly.[9] But what are similar situations? If the basis of egalitarianism—our fundamental equality as persons—is stressed, then it would seem that everyone is similarly situated and identical treatment is required. But if the main goal of egalitarianism—respect for persons—is stressed, then it would seem that our individual needs as persons must be addressed, and dissimilar treatment is required in order to attain similar results. And in either case, there is an additional practical issue. On the one hand, how can persons be treated identically, given the diversity of their situations and needs? On the other hand, how can these diverse individual situations and needs be understood or measured with sufficient accuracy in order to tailor treatments specifically designed to result in equal satisfactions?

The second problem with egalitarianism has to do with its difficulty in handling claims of individual merit, or desert. If the basis of egalitarianism lies not in any empirical assessment of individual persons' real accomplishments (an assessment sure to be widely unequal), but in an estimate of persons' equal dignity, it would seem that the theory cannot admit individual claims of unequal treatment based on merit. To claim to deserve something is to appeal to a particular empirical achievement or status. Egalitarianism cannot easily countenance such special pleading. But these considerations seem also to be part of our intuitive sense of justice. Does it not seem right, for example, to give greater responsibilities and the rewards that go with them to those with greater talent? Is it not intuitively unjust to give someone who works harder the same salary as everyone else? These are difficult issues for egalitarianism because both the talented and the untalented, the hard working and the lazy are equally valuable persons, considered simply as persons.

Finally, a general problem with egalitarianism is its lack of fit with the empirical world of inequalities. Part of our practical self-respect comes from our belief that we are different from and therefore unequal (that is, superior) to others in many ways.[10] The American economy depends on and in part glories in the inequalities of persons' situations. To what extent can a commitment to equality fit with these other realities? How equal, for example, must general circumstances be for equal rights to be meaningful claims? And if a far more thoroughgoing empirical equality of people is called for in order to realize the promise of equal human rights, how practical a project is this? More important, how compatible is a generalized commitment to egalitarianism with other important human values, such as freedom, individuality, and efficiency.

These difficult problems with egalitarianism must be acknowledged in theory and in application. Still, this is a powerful moral framework. It accounts for much of our intuitive sense of justice and allows for development of a strong concept of human rights. It provides a foundation for a general understanding of the value of people. And it sets an agenda for reform in the direction of equal respect for all intrinsically and incalculably valuable persons.

Substantive equality

It would appear that a right to health care follows naturally from the implications of egalitarianism for human rights. This is probably the case. But lest this conclusion be drawn too quickly, a major objection to guaranteeing entitlement to health care on egalitarian grounds must be considered.

It might be argued that establishing a right to health care in a market economy actually has antiegalitarian implications because it would involve taking some resources from some—by taxation, for example—and returning them to others—in the services that would be guaranteed. This is unequal treatment on its face. Alternatively, leaving the distribution of health care wholly to the marketplace is the genuinely egalitarian solution, since everyone is treated (or not treated) equally: all are free to purchase whatever health care they can afford.

A reply to this objection must begin by appealing to the distinction between procedural and substantive equality, between equality measured by similarity of treatment and by similarity of result. Surely, the objection is accurate insofar as a guarantee of entitlement to health care would probably redistribute resources, taking from some and giving to others. Since this means treating persons differently, a right to health care would have to embody more of a substantive egalitarianism than a procedural egalitarianism. The justification for this bias is obvious. The very nature of health care is predicated on the existence of human needs, universal but unequal human needs, for the prevention and treatment of conditions that cause pain, suffering, disability, and premature death.[11] The very motive for providing health care and claiming a right of access to it relies on the fact of these needs and so must incline toward substantive, or result-oriented, egalitarianism. If we presume that similar treatment for similar cases entails providing health care for those in need of it but not for those without the need, then a meaningful right to health care in an unequal social environment must rely on the transfer of resources from the healthy and well-off to the ill and poor. In terms of the main goal of egalitarianism, respect for all persons, this seems to be a reasonable transfer. Add to the equation that those who are now healthy will one day be (or have been) ill and in need of health care, and the transfer seems even more reasonable.

In this light, the equality attained by the marketplace is illusory. When everyone is equally free to purchase health care in the marketplace, but some do not have the private resources to afford even the most basic care, then procedural equality masks the production of avoidable human suffering, which is obviously incompatible with a substantive moral mandate to respect persons. In a market economy such as ours, with its large inequalities of income and without entitlement to health care, the purchase of insurance and the use of preventive care, including care for fetuses, children, and all those dependent on others, are deferred in favor of the purchase of goods and services that satisfy other needs thought to be more pressing. Early, economical, and effective treatment is delayed until treatment is urgent, more expensive, and less likely to succeed. The empirical consequences of this market approach have been described in Chapter 1. The health care system is misused, the emergency room playing the role of the unavailable primary care, for example. And many bona fide health care needs simply go unmet. It understates the conclusion significantly to say that this adds up to a considerable amount of unnecessary pain, suffering, disability, and premature death for intrinsically and incalculably valuable persons. From the egalitarian viewpoint presented here, such a result is a violation of a fundamental human right, the right to respect for persons' bodies and minds.

Another basis for the claim of a right to health care follows from the fundamental political rights that egalitarianism wants to ensure. Guaranteeing entitlement to health care would protect equality of opportunity by helping those disadvantaged by health status to participate more fully in life. Ensured access to health care regardless of ability to pay would promote equal personal liberty, allow more persons to construct and execute their own life plans, and permit more sharing in the control of institutions and policies that shape persons' lives. Certainly, all these opportunities are lost or compromised by serious health problems, many of which would be avoidable if there were guaranteed access to proper health care.

Finally, the right to health care can be seen to follow from the very basis of egalitarianism, respect for persons and its corollary of self-respect. A fundamental moral wrong is apparent in societies with gross inequalities.[12] The differences among persons are accentuated, to the detriment of those without a comparable share of those things and opportunities that the society affords to others. Meaningful and positive relationships among individuals from opposite ends of the opportunity spectrum become impossible. Interpersonal communication and the sense of community that it fosters suffer or are destroyed. Respect between persons at the extremes is attenuated. Thus the self-respect of those with graphically less is lost or never developed. This is patently the case in a slave society. But it can also be the case in a society of health care haves and have-nots. This is especially evident when the haves get access to the best care that our species has ever known and the have-nots get little or none. If the opportunity to develop self-respect is a basic human right, then compromising that opportunity through denial of needed health care or through provision of second-class care is a violation of a basic right.

Further light can be shed on the claim for a right to health care by comparing it with the other elements necessary for the cultivation of self-respect—the right to freedom from assault and the right to cultural literacy. The right to freedom from assault may at first seem distant from the right to health care. The former would seem to be a negative right of noninterference, whereas the latter is a positive right of access. But consider what a right to freedom from assault actually entails for a society that attempts to guarantee it.[13] Meaningful freedom from assault in an organized political society requires the establishment of a police force, with all the personnel, equipment, and buildings this involves. It also requires a judiciary and rights of access guaranteed to those assaulted and of proper protection of those accused of assault. This means judges, lawyers, courts, and other legal support. There must also be a way of punishing offenders. This means prisons, wardens, probation officers, and so on. The guarantee of this apparently negative right thus mandates large outlays of social resources. And there are clearly unequal needs in this area. Some citizens may never have recourse to the police and judiciary. Others—say, those who live or conduct businesses in high-crime areas—may absorb a great deal of the police and judiciary investment of a society. Yet these investments, supported by a transfer of resources from taxation to provision of services, are too clearly a matter of persons' fundamental rights to be left wholly to the marketplace.

The right to cultural literacy is an even closer analogue to the right to health care.[14] It is plain that a person who is denied effective access to symbols in a highly symbolic culture—say, one who was never taught to read in contemporary America—is a person whose intrinsic and incalculable value has not been respected by others. It is all too likely that in a society that presumes literacy, such a person will fail to develop an appropriate level of self-respect. But persons have a right to a level of education sufficient to permit a reasonably equal chance to develop self-respect and the respect of others. The guarantee of this right therefore mandates public investment in teachers and schools. And since the educational abilities of persons vary, their needs for special forms of education will vary as well. Society is obligated to transfer resources to satisfy this basic right.

A right to health care is a form of social protection, as is a right to freedom from assault; and it is a form of guaranteeing equitable access to a culture, as is a right to literacy. In all these cases, public investment of social resources must be made to ensure that people are respected for the values that they are. And in all these cases, substantive egalitarianism is the form of equality that makes more sense. It makes no sense, for example, to provide equal police surveillance in low-crime and high-crime areas; equal remedial-reading courses for all, whether or not they need them; equal health care for all, regardless of health status. Rather, each case calls for the unequal treatment of persons based on their unequal needs in order to make for a reasonable hope of equality of result for all. Thus a right to health care can be based on an egalitarian framework of respect for persons where that means a commitment to substantive rather than procedural equality.

There are probably a multitude of ways in which a society can establish systems to guarantee access to health care, just as there are a multitude of ways to organize police and educational systems. Substantive egalitarianism probably inclines toward one public system of health care delivery, since one system provides the best chance for an equal standard of care for those with similar needs throughout a whole society.[15] This might mean a government-operated national health service, but there are many models for structuring a system that is government regulated and financed but not government operated. At the other extreme, one can envision a system that includes a number of private or semiprivate health care providers, with the government's role restricted largely to that of financing health insurance or payment for the care in order to guarantee that no one's right to health care is compromised by inability to pay. The first alternative has the virtue of uniformity of service, but at the cost of increased government bureaucracy. The second has the virtue of more independent points at which to experiment with a diversity of services and settings, but at the likely cost of greater inequality of care. And a range of alternatives in between can be envisioned. The choice of which system is best is a prudential one affected by any number of variables, including comparable costs, efficiency, and the history and traditions of the society. But an egalitarian framework of respect for the intrinsic and incalculable value of persons leaves certain elements of a just health care system nonnegotiable: any acceptable system must provide substantively equal care to all in a context conducive to the development of persons' self-respect.

Further implications of an egalitarian basis for a right to health care can be made clear by considering the practical difficulties already identified with the theory. The first important issue turns on the nature of human needs. If we are to distribute resources in terms of needs, then we must be able to identify in practice the difference between a basic human need and a want or another sort of desire. This is a notoriously difficult task in any area, but especially so in health care.[16] We might start by describing as a basic human need those health care services that are necessary for the relief of pain and suffering and for the prevention of disabilities and premature death.[17] This is an intuitively plausible starting place because these are the general goals of health care, and by stating the goals negatively (relief of pain, not production of pleasure), some of the most extravagant health care claims can be eliminated. It cannot be the role of health care to provide for "complete physical, mental, and social well-being" for example, since this is an impossible goal to strive for and would expand the province of medicine into every aspect of human life.[18] But even put negatively, large problems of definition remain. It may be obvious on the basis of this interpretation of basic health care needs, for example, that a range of emergency services should be equally available, since they can demonstrably reduce the rate of premature deaths from accident. But should there be a right to a kidney transplant, a procedure medically and economically preferable to long-term dialysis, for which there is an existing legal right of reimbursement under Medicare?[19] No doubt, some level of basic prenatal care should be provided to all pregnant women and their fetuses. But should there be a right to in utero surgery to correct fetal defects? Suppose that such surgery were the only way to prevent brain damage from hydrocephalus or kidney damage from uropathy.[20] And who can say just where genuine health care ends and cosmetic treatment begins? Are contact lenses, face lifts, and hair transplants solely cosmetic? They appear to be in general, but they probably also relieve suffering in many cases. What if they were also shown to be associated with longer life; would they then be preventive of premature death and thereby covered by a right to health care?

Shot through these practical considerations is the economic question. Supposing that we could clarify the nature of basic health care sufficiently to answer some of the practical questions, can society afford every procedure and service for everyone who genuinely needs it? Suppose again, to dramatize the issue, that one individual needed the entire annual health care budget in order to prevent his or her premature death. Clearly, no system, regardless of its theoretical basis, could tolerate this kind of expenditure. Although exaggerated, the point is that even an egalitarian health care system based on respect for persons must limit the resources it commits. Under a private payer system, in which health care is not regarded as a right, but as a market commodity to be bought and sold like any other, the economic problem is not nearly so sharp. Because health care is not regarded as an entitlement, no violation of rights is involved when some persons are denied needed care because of their inability to pay for it. Perhaps a resultant premature death is unfortunate, even tragic, but outside the context of a right, there is no injustice in such a situation.[21] Once a commitment is made to guaranteeing a right to health care, however, the economic implications of guaranteeing that right become public and explicit. Furthermore, the motivation that leads an egalitarian to a right to health care, leads to claims for other rights. For example, public investments in education, housing, and the creation of jobs are probably just as necessary as health care in a society that respects persons. The economic demands of each of these needs have to be considered and weighed against those of health care.

Given these considerations, the egalitarian formula for the provision of basic health care would have to be adjusted to encompass what is not only necessary to relieve pain and suffering and to prevent disabilities and premature death, but also possible for a society to afford. Determining what the resources that a society could afford to spend on health care would require choices at two levels: allocating a certain reasonable proportion of total social resources to health care in general, and then allocating sums within the health care field itself. Both decisions would have to be animated by egalitarian commitments. The total level of health care spending would have to be justified by its comparative ability to contribute to equal respect for persons. If, for example, it could be shown that an investment in education has more impact on equalizing health characteristics than an investment in health care, this would be a strong argument in favor of spending comparatively more money for education and less for health care.[22] Clearly, such judgments are not made with precision or without a plainly political component. But as long as egalitarian principles are determinative of the outcome and persons have broadly equal access to society's political resources, imprecision and political decision making are not vitiating factors, but the necessary media for such public choices.

Within the field of health care itself, egalitarian distribution could proceed in one of three ways. The first option would be to exclude whole categories of patients from entitlement to some necessary but very expensive care.[23] For example, it might not be reasonable, certainly at this time, to guarantee entitlement to an artificial heart. The cost of supplying these hearts to all who need them would be prohibitively expensive. Rather than choosing who is entitled to get them and who is not, one egalitarian solution would be to deny that any of the candidates for artificial hearts are entitled to one. This policy would have the benefit of uniform treatment, but the drawback of providing no hearts to anyone when some might have been afforded. This policy of no treatment if all cannot be treated would also have a generally negative effect on health care innovation, since the early stages of the development of technologies are typically the most expensive and generally of initial benefit to a very few.

The second alternative would be to distribute care on the basis of fine-grained medical criteria for entitlement. Society might conclude, for example, that it can afford only 20 percent of the artificial-heart operations needed annually. It might then be acceptable to have a board of health care professionals screen candidates so that only those patients in the top 20 percent of prognoses for a successful implant would be selected. The criteria for successful outcomes would vary with the nature of the procedure and the state of health care technology. This screening would probably consider general state of health, presence or absence of secondary medical problems, and perhaps even pertinent psychological factors. Although this approach would allow some to be treated and would be more favorable to innovation, it would also be a more dangerous procedure for an egalitarian because untoward nonmedical factors might influence some decisions. It might, for example, lead to de facto discrimination against the elderly. Even if age were not used as a consideration, one can assume that past some age, the older a person is, the generally poorer the prognosis from such an operation. Still, one might reply that from the perspective of likely medical success, this policy would treat similarly situated persons similarly and thus is just from an egalitarian point of view.

The third egalitarian option could have elements of both the other approaches. If 20 percent of the needed operations could be afforded and some medical innovation were to be publicly encouraged, a random choice of 20 percent could be made from those with minimum medical qualifications.[24] That is, this approach would simply remove from consideration those for whom such an operation would be of no reasonable benefit, and then select by lot from the remaining pool of candidates the 20 percent to receive the operation. Random choice respects everyone equally, since all have an equal chance to be selected.

Note that none of these three options truly guarantees an entitlement to either identical treatment, as would be mandated by a strict interpretation of procedural equality, or to identical results, as would be mandated by a strict interpretation of substantive equality. Strict procedural equality must be abandoned because the delivery of health care arises out of an unequally distributed need. Strict substantive equality must also be abandoned because no society's resources could ever be such that it could guarantee entitlement to health care sufficient to secure equal freedom from pain, suffering, disability, and premature death for all. But by using both principles together, a reasonable egalitarian right to health care can be described. First, persons have an equal entitlement to needed basic health care to the degree that society can afford to provide it. Second, the determination of what is basic and what society can afford is to be made in a political process to which all have relatively equal access (a vote, ability to organize, access to elected officials) and which is dominated by the twin concerns of achieving substantive equality in the funding of health care in general and achieving procedural equality in the distribution of resources earmarked for health care. In short, we begin with unequal human needs and tailor society's ability to address these needs on the basis of treating similar cases similarly.

The second general problem with egalitarianism has to do with desert. How are we to treat voluntary high-risk takers—for example, helmetless motorcyclists, cigarette smokers, sky divers, those who never exercise? It does not seem right that those who knowingly expose themselves to greater risks to their health should have their behavior subsidized by those who take reasonable steps to avoid injury and prevent sickness. In other words, should not a just health care system recognize and reward health-related desert? But if so, an egalitarian system of health care is not just. Such a system not only fails to recognize desert in those who try to preserve their health, but may actually encourage irresponsibility by distributing care on the basis of need, a principle of distribution sure to favor those who take less care of their own health.[25]

Several responses are possible. First, there is no reason why an egalitarian system of health care could not acknowledge desert to some extent.[26] It would be acceptable to levy a health care tax on cigarettes, alcohol, and high-cholesterol foods, for example, and to divert that money toward helping to pay for the care of those with diseases caused by the use of these products. Special fees for health care could be placed on dangerous activities, such as taking ski lifts and carnival rides, and extra fees levied on the purchase of cars, boats, planes, and motorcyles. Society could correspondingly subsidize health-promoting activities through discounted fees for programs to stop smoking and drinking and for membership in fitness groups, or lower prices for fruits and vegetables known to promote health. Such fees and discounts would help shift some health costs in line with desert and would provide incentives for health-promoting behavior.

But such attempts to accommodate desert can go only so far, given a general commitment to egalitarianism's respect for persons. Society could not, for example, refuse to provide care to the victim of lung cancer or a motorcycle accident. An egalitarian right to health care would have to reject such an extreme desert-based view for three reasons.[27] First, we will likely never have the kind of grasp of causation necessary to make the individual judgments that a desert-based view would require. Although we may know that on any reasonable interpretation of causation, long-term cigarette smoking causes lung cancer, can we know that a particular individual's own smoking caused his cancer? Can we rule out the causal effects of ambient pollution for which this individual is not responsible, of childhood X-rays authorized by uninformed parents, or of genetic predispositions in general? We may know that as a rule, riding a motorcycle without a helmet is an exceptionally dangerous activity, but can we know in this case that the accident was not the other driver's fault? Supposing that the injured motor-cyclist was only partly to blame, would the degree of care be proportioned to the degree of responsibility, and how could we determine these degrees? What if the motorcylist was on a bona fide emergency, and the helmet that she otherwise always wears had been stolen? To how much care would she be entitled?

Second, we are equally far from an understanding of free choice, which would be needed to assign responsibilities in a desert-based system. Is cigarette smoking, for example, a choice or an addiction? If the answer is that it is an addiction born of choice, were those first choices free— uncoerced by teen-age peer pressure, for example? Were the choices in-formed; that is, did the smoker understand the implication of those early choices at the time of the choices? Can we ignore other known psychosocial determinants of such a choice: the ubiquity of slick, subliminally seductive advertisements; government subsidies for the growing and processing of tobacco, familiar class-based and regional patterns of behavior among others? And what if there are underlying genetic predispositions to nicotine addiction, as there appear to be with alcoholism and obesity? In sum, our inability in specific cases to unravel the complexities of freedom and deter-minism in a manner that is fair to someone who, by hypothesis, is already suffering from a health care need makes a desert-based delivery system untenable in theory.

Finally, such a proposal would be unworkable in practice. Even if we could sort out the causal and choice-related factors in principle, could we do it instantly and reliably at the door of a hospital emergency room? Would we want to place that burden on health care professionals? Could they maintain a general stance of sympathy toward the sick and injured if they were asked to be so judgmental? Could society as a whole do so? Would we not be blaming persons who were already victims of injury and disease?

The third problem with an egalitarian basis for a right to health care concerns the tension between demanding equality in health care while accepting widespread inequalities in other important areas of life, especially in the distribution of such other basic necessities as food and shelter. A point made earlier is appropriate again. From an egalitarian perspective, there should be more equality in life generally, and most especially in access to life's necessities. But even among the basic human needs, health care stands out as requiring special attention. As noted already, the need for health care is often overriding when it occurs and is unequally distributed, and the patient is in an exceptionally dependent position vis-à-vis the health care professional. Equally important from the egalitarian point of view is the potent effect of health care on the development of self-respect, for better or worse. Health care's directly personal character, its intimacy in the revelation of private bodily and mental experiences, and the awesome nature of the encounter with technology that it allows converge to make the health care exchange a context in which persons' self-respect can be uniquely enhanced or diminished. Compare, for example, the impact on self-respect of a therapeutic encounter in a doctor's office between a suburban professional and the familiar family doctor with the impact of an encounter in an emergency room of an inner-city hospital between an unknown foreign-born medical resident and an individual piece of human "teaching materials."[28] Thus even if American society resists a general commitment to greater equality, a separate argument exists for it with respect to health care.

Also related to the general inequality of our society is the question of whether to permit the purchase of health care outside the egalitarian public system that the government would likely operate or finance. There are some good reasons not to permit this.[29] Obviously, the possibility of buying care in place of or in addition to that provided by a public system would compromise some of the equality otherwise guaranteed by the public system. Alternative delivery systems would likely cater largely to those able to pay more—that is, the generally well off—and thus might create a drain of talent and other health care resources out of a public system. Additionally, putting everyone into one public system would serve to elevate the overall quality of care in the system, since the rich and powerful would be served there too. Their own self-interest and that of their families would be best served by ensuring the highest affordable quality in the public system. Finally, if too many members of the middle class were able to join the rich in purchasing health care outside the public system, that system would tend to lose its critical mass and become more of a welfare system of health care for the poor. The likely implication of this is public hostility, chronic underfunding, and a deteriorated, demoralized system. By contrast, a high-quality public system for all might be a source of civic pride and a focus for national unity.

But there are also strong arguments against prohibiting alternatives. First, there is at least an irony in forbidding the rich from buying additional, perhaps needed health care, while permitting the free purchase of luxury items. We allow the purchase of private alternatives and supplements to other socially provided necessities: private education and the services of private security guards, for example. More to the heart of the matter, there must always be a bias against prohibiting free access to goods or services in any free society, and there is probably a strong one in place in contemporary American society. Practically, it is difficult to see how such a prohibition could be enforced without compromising other important values. Would we prohibit travel to a foreign country to buy health care services, for example?[30] Additionally, part of the vitality of the American health care system to date is based on its pluralistic character, including the historical and present contributions of many voluntary and religiously based hospitals and health care–delivery systems. This has contributed to the variety and innovative character of American medicine, and it might well be lost were a public system mandated for all.

Perhaps a middle way can be found between these alternatives. A public health care system could be legally protected against some kinds of competition from private alternatives, as are some public utilities, so that it would retain a core of public use and support, while a certain range of options would be permitted outside the system. The balance could be reset politically as needed, with the goal of ensuring both a strong and high-quality public health care system and a reasonable range of freedom and innovation outside the system. At this point, philosophical speculation must simply defer to common sense and a society's traditions.

A final problem with an egalitarian health care system in a nonegalitarian society should be noted. It may be objected that it is simply unacceptably paternalistic to design a public system to solve problems that individuals could or should try to solve for themselves. To raise resources by taxation in order to provide health care services is an act of paternalism: the imposition of choices on adults for their (alleged) own good whether or not they agree with those choices for themselves. But there are two good responses to this charge of paternalism. First, many of those who now suffer from the failings of the American health care system are not competent adults, but fetuses, children, and incompetent adults. Providing health care for these groups either is not paternalism or is morally justified paternalism. Second, and perhaps more fundamentally, the construction of institutions to provide public services is a legitimate moral and political choice for a democratic community of adults to make.[31] As long as individuals have some range of alternatives outside the public system and, more important, as long as we protect the fundamental moral right of adults to informed consent over their own health care, including the implied right to refuse treatment, government action on behalf of an egalitarian right to health care will not be invidious paternalism. Construction of a public system of health care is thus no more inherently paternalistic than public provision of police protection and education. Such a democratic political choice would simply be an institutional response to genuine human needs based on an appraisal of each person as intrinsically and incalculably valuable.

5

Libertarianism

Egalitarianism depends ultimately on viewing the individual person as a being of intrinsic and incalculable value. As we have seen, a very strong case for a right to health care can be made by starting with that presumption about persons. But a similar starting place with a change of emphasis results in another perspective, from which claims about a positive right to health care are not only invalid, but also dangerous. That perspective is libertarianism.

Persons are beings of intrinsic and incalculable value because they value other beings. In order to value something, it must be understood to some extent; at the very least, it must be recognized. The highest human expression of the understanding crucial to having values is rationality. Rationality, briefly, is the ability to consider various aspects of anything, real or imagined; to compose plans of real or imagined action; and to relate various realities or imagined realities to one another in order to discover or construct coherence and meaningfulness. In short, rationality is the ability to think, to plan, to appraise.

To be in a position to value someone or something requires more than rationality, however. It also requires choice. In the very process of thinking, there is already appraisal, the tendency to like or dislike, to select or reject. Sometimes this is tacit, as in the usual development of a taste or distaste for certain colors or foods. Sometimes it is explicit, as in deliberations about career or marriage. In either case and in all those in the great space in between, to think is also to judge and therefore to begin to choose.

Taken together, the abilities to think and to choose allow humans to be rational agents—that is, autonomous, self-determining beings.[1] And this characteristic of persons, perhaps more than any other, is what constitutes human freedom. Because they can think, persons can understand their circumstances and the alternatives available to them. Because they can choose, persons can act to affirm or change their circumstances. Because they can think and choose, persons are free to create their own life plans and the values of which they are made.

Liberty and ownership

Emphasis on persons' freedom as rational agents is at the core of libertarianism.[2] From this perspective, the fundamental right of persons is to have their rational agency respected. The greatest threat to rational agency comes from the use of coercion to restrict individuals' liberty to think and choose for themselves. Violence and threats of violence, theft, fraud, and breach of promise undermine rational agency and, with it, personal liberty.[3] They are thus violations of persons' rights, compromises of what persons are inherently entitled to. These coercions are wrong, even if they should result in greater happiness or greater equality for persons. They are wrong because they undermine respect for persons. Persons have both a right of individual liberty and a corresponding duty not to interfere with the liberty of others regardless of the consequences.

Because it is grounded in the fundamental right of personal liberty, the duty not to interfere with others' rational agency is the strongest moral obligation. This strong obligation acts as a constraint on all other moral values.[4] It forbids the imposition of any form of coercion on rational adults. Other moral values, such as producing happiness or achieving greater equality of opportunity, can be sought only insofar as they do not violate the fundamental right of personal liberty. Thus if these other moral values generate obligations, they must be weaker than the obligation of noninterference. If, for example, there is a general duty to aid others in distress, it is constrained by the duty not to interfere with anyone's liberty in doing so. The latter duty is founded in a fundamental right, and therefore its violation would be outright unjust. To fail to aid the distressed, by contrast, would not violate a fundamental right, since only liberty is a fundamental right. Thus the failure to aid may be unkind, inhumane, or lacking from any number of other moral perspectives, but it is not unjust. We may well have duties to aid those in distress; it is not part of the project of libertarianism to deny the richness and complexity of moral obligation. But whatever those duties are, they arise out of concerns for charity, not for justice.[5]

Another way to put this point is with the language of negative and positive rights. For the libertarian, the only true rights, the only primary entitlements that must be socially guaranteed, are negative rights of noninterference. The most familiar rights in American political experience are of this sort. Rights to freedom of speech, religion, and assembly are rights to be free from coercion by others, especially the government. The so-called positive rights of access—rights to education, employment, housing, and a decent standard of living—are not rights at all for the libertarian, but are manifesto assertions of desiderata.

But these manifesto claims for positive rights are more than empty. They are also dangerous. In every case, these alleged rights can be satisfied only by the violation of someone else's real negative rights. It is characteristic of negative rights generally that they can be universally satisfied when everyone does nothing. A person's right to freedom of speech is satisfied as long as no one does anything to abridge it; universal nonaction suffices. But so-called positive rights require that a person be provided access to some goods or services by society. These goods and services must come from somewhere. In most cases, the private resources of some people must be taken by the government in the form of taxes to pay for others' access to these goods and services. Taxation, of course, is a coercive taking, as witnessed by the penalties imposed for tax evasion. Therefore, in most cases, claims for positive rights of access can be satisfied only by the government's taking of private resources. But the use of coercion violates the fundamental right of personal liberty. Thus positive rights can be had only by violating negative rights. But since negative rights are grounded in the fundamental right of personal liberty, they may not be violated. Therefore, there can be no positive rights.[6]

It is plain from its rejection of positive rights that libertarianism puts great stress on the protection of persons' ownership of property in the form of both goods and services. On this account, personal liberty is violated not only when a person is interfered with directly, but also when the rightful possessions of a person are coercively taken. Ownership is important because persons invest their rational choices in their property, through their care for their goods and their labor to develop service skills, for example. Possessions thus become extensions of their owners. Furthermore, property is a powerful means of protecting and enhancing one's range of rational choice, of ensuring self-determination. Where theft, fraud, or breach of contract prevail, no guarantee of rational choice is possible. But most of all, the failure to protect ownership makes persons constantly vulnerable to coercion and threats of coercion through their property. Second only to the negative right of personal noninterference and closely related to it is the negative right of noninterference with personal property.[7]

In terms of the example of distributing employee health care benefits, the libertarian approach would be to establish ownership of the benefits first. If the owners of the company possess these resources justly and have no contracts with or have made no promises to their employees, no further questions of rights are at issue. They may distribute the benefits in any way or no way at all without violating any of the employees' rights. None of them has a right to the health care benefits because none of them owns them, and there are no positive rights of access to what is not owned.

It is also clear that a theory of the role of government is implied here. For libertarianism, the government's main legitimate function is to provide for the protection of negative rights—that is, to establish a framework for justice. It must therefore provide for defense from threat of extranational violence, maintain an internal police force to prevent the use of coercion by one citizen against another, and construct and enforce laws against theft, fraud, and breach of contract. Closely related is the government's responsibility to rectify injustice. It must provide a general mechanism for the peaceful resolution of disputes, punish violators, and provide redress for those whose rights have been violated, including compensation for possessions unjustly taken by others. This is a description of the minimal state.[8] Among the activities it may not engage in are any attempts to coerce citizens into the redistribution of private resources in order to achieve any preferred pattern of holdings. While such redistribution may serve many important moral goals, including increasing happiness, producing greater equality among persons, and aiding the needy, these goals are not legitimately pursued by the state. Individual or collective voluntary efforts to achieve these goals are acceptable. They may even be mandatory for libertarianism, if they follow from duties of charity, for example. But duties of charity do not give rise to rights that can be claimed by the recipients of the charity.[9] Thus they can make no rightful demand on the government that it use its coercive power on their behalf. Instead, the government is bound in justice to refrain from wrongfully taking what is owned by others and must use its coercive power to see that others refrain as well.

Justice, then, simply is respecting persons and what they rightfully own. Outside the range of governmental action, persons may rightfully come to own goods or service skills in one of two general ways.[10] First, the possession may have been originally unowned, and the present owner acquired it properly. In the case of land or an unowned natural resource, this involves taking the object and combining one's labor with it in such a way as to create an enhanced value without substantially precluding the ability of others to do the same. This last qualification is not meant to apply to the general disadvantage caused to others merely by private ownership itself, since any private ownership creates the direct disadvantage that others cannot also possess what is privately owned. It is meant instead to exclude the possibility, say, of acquiring the only well in an oasis for the purpose of denying water to others.[11] Short of extremes of this sort, virtually any act of initial acquisition adds value to a good by mixing it with the labor, however minor, of the owner and is thus just. The second way to come to own goods and services properly is to receive them through a just transfer. Land, for example, may be received as a gift from someone who owns it rightfully or through sale by exchange for anything else of value (money, goods, service, other land). As long as all parties agree to the transfer without violence, threat of violence, fraud, or breach of contract, it is by that fact just.

A third and final way to justly possess goods or services involves governmental action directly. If some holdings were acquired unjustly—through fraud, for example—or were transferred unjustly—by use of violence, for example—then the government is bound to rectify these injustices. Using its best historical information, the government must identify the individuals or the heirs of the individuals who unjustly gained these holdings and those who unjustly lost them and must redistribute the appropriate amount of resources from the first group to the second. This not only requires considerable historical knowledge, but also demands sophisticated subjunctive thinking—that is, deliberation on the patterns of ownership that might have resulted subsequent to just possession had the historical injustice not occurred.[12] Sometimes detailed historical knowledge will be lacking or subjunctive reasoning will yield too many alternatives of what might have been. When this is the case and when the injustice is thought to have been large and systematic, it may be necessary for the government to merely select a plausible rule to guide a wholesale redistribution from those who most likely benefited from past injustices to those who most likely were harmed by them. For example, one might assume that in a situation of large-scale injustice, the historical victims of injustice, although nameless, generally were made worse off because of it. Furthermore, since advantages and disadvantages tend to accrue over generations, the worst-off in present-day society probably include a great number of the descendents of those who were harmed by injustice in the past. Then the government might have to adopt a rectifying rule of thumb, such as "organize society so as to maximize the position of whatever group ends up least well-off in the society."[13] A rule of this sort offers the greatest likelihood of ensuring that victims of injustice and their descendents receive some of the compensation they deserve. Still, it must be recalled that for libertarianism, commitment to the use of any such redistributive rule is not called for by the nature of justice itself, but by the requirement that government rectify past injustice.

As a consequence, a just arrangement of ownership in society is not based on maximizing happiness, equalizing self-respect, recognizing merit, or acknowledging any other material, result-oriented principle. A just arrangement is any arrangement of ownership of property acquired and transferred justly. The sole legitimate interest of government in the distribution of property, therefore, is to ensure that it is acquired and transferred justly. Because there will inevitably be injustice, the government must also establish a means of restoring property or otherwise providing compensation to those who have unjustly lost what they owned. But on the libertarian account, if goods and services are held justly, it is not the business of government to select some preferred pattern of property ownership and redistribute resources in that direction. Although it may be disguised as a form of taxation, government redistribution, whether outright or in the form of social and welfare services, to achieve some preferred pattern, is a coercive taking of justly held personal resources. To those whose income is derived primarily from their labor, taxation for redistribution to others is a form of forced labor.[14]

This may seem to be an insensitive conclusion in the face of the great suffering caused by the inequities in the distribution of American health care. But again, the libertarian need not deny an obligation in charity to help redistribute resources voluntarily. The theory must, however, place a priority on personal liberty as the fundamental human right. From this perspective, claims for positive rights and the demand that government coercively tax private resources to fund such rights are derived not from justice, but from the psychology of envy.[15] Envy is a self-defeating disposition because it leads to the evaluation of one's own worth by comparison with what others have. The envious thus prefer that all have the same or that all have nothing and refuse to allow some to have more, even if this more is received justly. In their demand for equality, the envious will use the state to interfere more and more in persons' lives and property in order to equalize. This will substantially diminish the pluralism of society. The artificial equalization of persons will necessitate the curtailment of the free exchange of values between rational agents and thus entail a loss of variety, innovation, risk taking, and efficiency. Through this leveling process, power will come to be centralized in the state. But the worst consequence of the attempt to equalize is the threat that it represents to the central importance of human persons: it undermines rational agency and the personal liberty it sustains.

Libertarianism is an important ethical perspective, and its warnings about compromising individual liberty and fostering the growth of the state are surely important lessons. But there are substantial theoretical difficulties with libertarianism. First, there are problems in trying to distinguish strongly between negative and positive rights and between a minimal and a redistributive state. In order to accomplish the goals of even the most minimal of states, funds must be invested in the military, police, courts, prisons, regulators of fraud, and other order-enforcement agencies. This is hardly inaction and noninterference. Instead, the logic of effective social guarantee of noninterference demands that a great deal be done by the government. These functions must be paid for by taxes levied on private resources, and they will often have redistributive effects. Some parts of a country may be more in need of defense from foreign attack; some may benefit more from military installations and armament contracts. Some people have greater need for police because they have more to protect or because they live and do business in high-crime areas. If those victimized by fraud and breach of contract are to have their grievances redressed, they must be guaranteed positive access to courts, judges, and lawyers who will see to it that their negative rights are upheld. But if all are taxed at the same or similar rate and use these services disproportionately, then redistribution of resources is the result. The implication of these considerations is that the distinction between negative and positive rights and between a minimal and a redistributive state may not be as sharp as libertarianism supposes.[16]

Second, it seems intuitively wrong to say that justice has nothing to do with persons' happiness or suffering, with the relative distribution of resources in a society, or with merit. The claim that social justice lies only in the history of justice in individual acquisitions and transfers seems overdrawn. It is certainly at odds with the great studies of justice done in the West, virtually all of which assume that some factors in the resulting pattern of ownership in a society at least contribute to an appraisal of that society as just or unjust. Imagine, for example, a society in which 90 percent of the population works exceptionally hard but nonetheless suffers from chronic grinding poverty and the other 10 percent does nothing but enjoy boundless opulence. Suppose that the 10 percent are descendents of persons who initially acquired their wealth justly, according to the libertarian model, and whose generations of well-born descendents transferred the wealth justly. Must we say that the situation is just because of this history? Is there no amount of suffering or inequality that is unjust on its face?

Third, the libertarian perspective systematically ignores certain positive externalities, the contributions that society makes to the welfare of all individuals. The ability of any individual to make rational choices and to acquire and transfer goods and services is set in a social context.[17] Rationality requires not only personal thought, but also the social tools of language and logic. Choice requires not only individual effort, but also traditions and socialization into habits of choice. Acquisition and transfer of resources requires not only police, but also a cultural framework in which individual possession makes sense and a network of inherited customs, laws, and technology. In short, libertarianism is an extreme form of individualism that overlooks the individual's real debts to persons who came before, to those who share the world of the present, and to the institutional realities created by the patterns of these persons' interactions. Society is very much a collective achievement, and to the extent that libertarianism ignores this social reality, it is an inadequate moral framework.

Fourth, the libertarian theory of justice in original acquisition is speculative beyond application in general, and where it can be applied at all, it tends to demonstrate the injustice of entire societies. Who can say whether the structure of ownership in present-day France, for example, is just, if this judgment requires an account of the original acquisition of French property. Who in fact originally acquired property in what is now France is shrouded forever in lost ancient societies. The likeliest guess, based on the history of known invasions and conquests, is that "original" possession was made and maintained by force. If this is so, every subsequent transfer of property has been infected by these original injustices. In nations whose written history is shorter, such as the United States, original possession by Native Americans was not individual ownership of the sort envisioned by libertarianism. Much of the subsequent "original" personal possession by Europeans was accomplished by force or deception, again tainting every state of possession since then with these original injustices. Should the libertarian conclusion be that all present possession in France and the United States is unjust? If so, what should be done, and who should be compensated? What subjunctive deliberations are appropriate or even possible? Should all property in France and the United States simply be redistributed to improve the positions of the least well-off in both nations? Since it is unlikely that libertarianism could countenance the implications of what appears on the basis of its own principles to be massive systematic injustice, defenders of the view would probably have to reject these considerations and simply presume that most original acquisitions were just. Or they might invoke a (morally arbitrary) statute-of-limitations scheme, whereby an injustice can no longer be rectified after some fixed time period. Then the opposite, equally unacceptable, result follows: the theory moves toward a wholesale justification of the status quo.

One might object to the very first presumption of this theory of just acquisition—that unowned nature is available for private taking and that combining labor with nature creates a fundamental right of private property. One could as easily make the opposite and equally plausible presumption (equal because neither can be proved) that nature is a common possession of all persons and no fundamental right of private ownership exists. On this presumption, the private possession of parts of commonly held nature is either unjustified theft or a practical arrangement justified only to the extent that it serves the common good from which it derives. In these cases, some form of compensation or return of benefits to society from the possessors of private property would be required by justice.[18]

The last theoretical problem with libertarianism is its overly sanguine presumptions about the contexts of the transfer of value. Even if the threats of force, fraud, and breach of contract were wholly eliminated, the inequality of persons' starting positions makes for inequality in bargaining position at the point of negotiating the terms of a transfer. Those beginning with wealth and its associated advantages are more than a match for those with little or nothing at the bargaining table. Assuming, for illustration, that we could begin with just acquisitions and that these initial just starts were broadly equal, it is still likely that over generations some would amass more than others through accident, effort, or both. When persons acquire significant resources, they typically advantage their offspring with them through inheritance. So the affluent will keep inheriting money with which to invest and make more money, while the poor will inherit less or nothing. That the poor will eventually have their rational choices controlled by circumstances systematically favoring the wealthy is neither surmise nor an expression of envy; it is the lesson of history. In short, even on the assumption of equal starting points and without presuming injustice in transfer, the protection of transfer itself, without concern for the results of transfer, can produce what seems to be injustice. But libertarianism cannot judge it so. When these ideal presumptions are put aside for reality, the situation for libertarian theory is worse yet. Persons did not, they do not, start equally. The historical contexts of original acquisition and subsequent transfer have been filled with violence (including slavery), threat of violence, theft, and every other form of injustice. How are we in the present to sort out which of the resulting possessions are justly held and which are too thoroughly compromised by historical injustices in both acquisition and transfer? That libertarianism can provide no guidance on this crucial question of the practical application of its own principles is its final major flaw.

Compensatory rights

Given the theoretical commitments of libertarianism, it is easy to see that any claim for a positive right to health care must be rejected.[19] To guarantee such an entitlement would entail the coercive taking of what is owned by others, and hence would involve a violation of the fundamental right of noninterference. There may still be a duty to aid those in need of health care, but this duty arises out of charity and not justice.

Libertarianism is quite compatible with a negative right in this context, however, a right of health noninterference.[20] Certainly, if the range of protected personal liberty extends as far as the things one owns, it would have to include one's state of physical and mental health as well. Mental health is too intimately associated with rational agency to be excluded from protection by right on the libertarian account.

A right of health noninterference would mean a right of freedom from actions by others that diminish a person's state of health. Just as homicide, the ultimate and irreversible violence against rational choice, would have to be illegal in a libertarian society, so would intentional infliction with a deadly disease. The police power of the state would have to be employed against such a violation of fundamental right. Negligent infliction of health harms would have to be illegal, too, just as negligent infliction of other harms is in the law of torts. In a libertarian society, one could sue to recover damages based on diminished health caused by a negligently manufactured consumer product, for example. Part of the legitimate function of even a minimal state is compensation for injustice, and it is surely a form of fraud or breach of contract to be sold a dangerous product without warning. Suits against environmental polluters would also have to be included, subject, of course, to the same standards of proof in causation as prevail in other areas of personal-injury law. Wrongful injury on the job, on public transportation, or as the result of anyone else's intentional or negligent act of commission or omission would be included. Malpractice awards for injury to health due to a health professional's incompetent performance or advice would be recoverable. Claims could also be made against the government itself, if its activities had a negative health impact on individuals. And harms to mental health, perhaps the most damaging from the perspective of rational agency, would merit compensation as well. Obviously, guaranteeing even this negative right to health noninterference would require considerable public investment in police, courts, lawyers, prisons, and other governmental agencies.

But it is also important to see what would not be covered by a libertarian right of health noninterference. In all the examples just cited, no real health care would be secured, unless it were specified as part of the monetary award of a court or jury in a personal-injury trial or agreed to by the parties as a settlement to avoid trial. In most cases, intentional health violators would be punished and negligent violators made to compensate their victims monetarily, but no access to health care would be made available directly. Furthermore, all these cases rely on the assignment of responsibility for someone's diminished health on some other person or institution. If an individual's health were diminished but no one were clearly responsible, there would be no guaranteed access even to the money that might be used to purchase health care and certainly none to health care itself. In cases of injury, illness, and incapacity due to faultless accident, disease, birth with genetic defect, old age, and the like, there is no right of access to health care on the libertarian account. These cases, of course, make up the greater part of contemporary health care. In addition, although libertarianism allows for compensation after damage to health as a right, it cannot accept preventive health care as a right. One is personally free to buy any and all kinds of health care. But there is no right to it.

What is omitted in this approach is the distribution of health care based on need. For libertarianism, positive access to health care follows only from ownership: health care services are some sort of original possession, are purchased through a rational and free choice to transfer something else of value in exchange for them, or are gained as compensation for past injustice. The only remaining avenue of access to care is charity—health care transferred to the recipient as a gift. Just as happiness and equality are theoretically irrelevant for determining the justice of a libertarian society, so are persons' needs in determining the just distribution of health care. Any pattern of distribution of health care might be just: no health care at all, health care for 10 percent and not for 90 percent or for 90 percent and not for 10 percent, for the employed but not the unemployed, for the wealthy but not the poor, even for the well but not the sick. Literally, any pattern resulting from just acquisition, transfer, and compensation is by that fact just.

One might object that this is plainly irrational, that the very point of providing health care is to meet the human need for it.[21] A society that allows the affluent ready access to cosmetic face lifts, for example, but the poor, no access to prenatal care seems to be missing the very purpose of health care. Care and need for the care, the objection might proceed, are logical correlates; they naturally go together, the latter justifying the former. Furthermore, to deny a right to health care is to allow a continuing compromise of the ability of the sick and incapacitated to enjoy a full range of rational choice. Those who die prematurely are cut off from rational choice entirely. This loss of rational choice because of lack of health care shows that 'the need for health care is basic and that a positive right to it is fundamental.

The libertarian response to this objection is direct, however. Because there exists a certain natural or logical relationship between two activities does not create a right to coerce persons into supporting one or both of the activities. Assertions about the natural and logical connection between health care and the need for it are theoretical. Real connections between them must be made by individuals' rational choices. If individuals judge the connection to be natural and logical, they will choose to devote their own resources and energies to see that their needs are met. This ensures a pluralism of interpretation of just what is natural and logical. Moreover, persons have a variety of needs. What needs are basic is a matter of considerable disagreement. If behavior is used as evidence, some persons judge access to health care to be important, and some do not. Some persons invest their private resources in it, in health insurance and preventive activities, for example. Others choose to buy less or no insurance so that they can invest their resources elsewhere, and they do not take measures to avoid illness and injury. The claim that health care is a logical response to a basic need runs counter to this evidence. Since guaranteeing a right to health care would probably mean forcing a health care investment (through taxes) on some who evidently do not value it enough to make the investment themselves, establishing a right to health care is unacceptably paternalistic. It imposes an alleged good on rational persons and thereby preempts their own choices.

More important perhaps than the imposition on the taxpayers who would have to purchase a social service that they may not want is the potential compromise of the liberty of health care professionals that the guarantee of a right to health care might entail. Health care professionals acquire their knowledge and skills by their own efforts and by the transfer of some of their private resources. With these competences, they provide health care on the basis of the rational choices of others to exchange values with them for it. Their position is therefore the same as others: personal liberty allows for acquisition and transfer on the basis of their own rational choices. But to create a right to health care would threaten that position. If there were a social guarantee of entitlement to health care, someone would have the duty to provide that care, but the only persons competent to do so would be trained health care professionals. Thus it appears that the only way to ensure a right to health care would be by coercing health care professionals to provide that care under circumstances that they did not and perhaps would not choose. This violates their fundamental liberty. The natural and logical connection between health care and the need for it should not disguise this violation any more than it would in other professions. There is a similar connection, for example, between the need for bread and the work of a baker and between the need for a haircut and the work of a barber.[22] In these cases, guaranteeing satisfaction of the need entails a compromise of the provider's personal freedom to choose whether and under what circumstances to transfer a service. Asserting a right to bread suggests a right to take what is owned by the baker. Asserting a right to a haircut suggests a right to take what is owned by the barber. But in both cases, there can be no such right because to effect it would mean to violate the fundamental right to personal liberty. So too in the case of health care: a right of access to health care means a violation of the liberty of providers.

For libertarianism, the question of need, while important from other moral perspectives, is simply irrelevant to the question of justice and rights in health care.[23] Suppose a situation of starvation: although we might say that the baker should give some bread to the hungry out of charity or even decency, would we say that the hungry have a right to the baker's bread? What would be the basis of their claim against the baker? Surely, the baker has what the hungry need, but many providers have goods and services that others need. We do not conclude from this that the needy have a right to what is not theirs simply because they need it. Health care needs stand out in this connection because they often have a dramatic and overriding character, but the structure of the human relationships at hand are the same. The mere existence of need does not justify taking what is needed from those who own it. Therefore, the simple fact of health care needs does not justify taking services from health care professionals. Again, there may be some very good moral reasons why these professionals and all citizens should strive voluntarily to meet others' health care needs. These moral reasons, however, are based on charity, and not on justice.

Some of these points can be brought together by considering what has been called the natural lottery.[24] All of us are born into circumstances not of our own choosing and beyond any use of the concept of desert. From a natural perspective, it appears to be a matter of pure fortune that some are born healthy, some ill; some into flush circumstances, some into deprivation; some have strong genetic resistance to disease, some are highly susceptible. Although we take increasing control over our lives as we mature, luck still plays a great role in life. Catching an airborne influenza or being injured by another's reckless driving, for example, appear to be largely matters of chance. Given that the way we start and a large part of what occurs afterward are governed by this natural lottery, what should our obligations in justice be toward the positions determined by the lottery? If no person can be assigned responsibility for the birth of a child with a genetic defect, for example, is the defect simply unfortunate, or is it also unjust?[25] Since it lies outside human control, how can it be unjust? And if it is not unjust, regardless of how tragic it is, can it be a duty in justice for anyone to have to provide care for the child's affliction? One might well argue that the child's parents bear some responsibility in justice, since their act brought the child into being. The libertarian could admit this. But do others have a duty and does the child have a corresponding right to needed health care? Surely, it would be praiseworthy if others chose to provide it. Some may even feel that it is incumbent on them because of personal religious or charitable commitments. But must they provide aid out of justice? The libertarian says no. Justice demands only that we respect personal liberty based on the moral centrality of human rational agency. It does not require that all needs be satisfied, even basic ones. And it outright prohibits their satisfaction with means that violate personal liberty.

The most inappropriate reaction to the natural lottery from the libertarian perspective is the demand for equality in access to health care. This demand is another expression of the psychology of envy. Just as the poor envy the circumstances of the wealthy, so the sick envy the circumstances of the well. The sick who are also poor envy the sick who are also wealthy because the wealthy can often purchase the kind of health care that will help them recover health or at least afford a greater range of care while sick. It is compatible with the psychology of envy that some who advocate an equal right to health care would rather have no one treated in some situations than allow access to only those who can afford to pay. The envious conclude this in spite of the fact that those who can afford to pay more may have justly received more or have chosen to invest more of what they have received into health care.

Although on this account the libertarian view is unalterably opposed to a positive right to health care in principle, there is a theoretical opening for a stronger response to health care needs than simply leaving their satisfaction to wholly voluntary efforts. A modified libertarian position can follow from further examination of the duty of charity.[26] Nothing in libertarianism opposes recognition of such a duty. Assume, then, that there is a duty to be charitable. Assume further that a libertarian society would be rational in its choices, willing and capable, that is, of matching effective means to desired goals. Such a society would be charitably concerned to meet the basic health care needs of citizens who could not afford to do so for themselves and concerned to develop an effective method to accomplish this goal. Suppose that private personal efforts to meet these needs were insufficient. Medicaid payments, one may assume, could not be replaced effectively by direct family-to-family giving. Suppose that even voluntary organizations relying on voluntary contributions did not suffice to address the needs. Perhaps this would be so because of the very high costs involved, the wide diversity of the needs, and the bureaucratic complexities of designing and delivering health care on a mass scale. The Red Cross, let us say, could not run the Veterans Administration effectively. If no voluntary system were capable of addressing the needs effectively, each person in a benevolent and rational libertarian society would have the charitable obligation to help and would genuinely want to help, but would also have a very good reason to do nothing: his or her individual contributions would be ineffective in a wholly voluntary system because there would be no guarantee that sufficient voluntary assistance from others would be forthcoming. Hence the charitable intent of any single person in a libertarian society would be frustrated. But if a government-operated or -financed system could rationally coordinate the discharge of the charitable duties of each citizen, then charity would be effective. In that case, the rational choice of all to be charitable could avoid frustration only if it were organized by a slightly more than minimal government. Rational and benevolent libertarians might therefore be inclined to accept this modification.

Such an arrangement would not constitute recognition of a right to health care because it would be a coordinated work of charity, not of justice. Since no rights would be at stake, there would be no standard for the care that must be provided other than that derived from the motive of charity itself. Thus no injustice would be done to those who received this care if it were less than all they needed or even if it were clearly inferior to the care that others were able to buy. It would be wholly up to the givers to determine the extent and the nature of their giving based only on their own standards of charity and decency. This modified libertarian approach is not just a thought experiment. Something very close to this reasoning persuaded the President's Commission for the Study of Ethical Problems in Medicine and Biomedical and Behavioral Research when in 1983 it wrote its report, *Securing Access to Health Care.*[27] The commission reached the conclusion that "society has a moral obligation to insure that everyone has access to adequate care" and that the government must guarantee this result, but also stated that there is no corresponding right to health care on the part of the recipients.[28] "For example," the commission wrote, "a person may have a moral obligation to help those in need, even though the needy cannot, strictly speaking, demand that person's aid as something they are due."[29]

Clearly, a pure libertarianism is inconsistent with this modified view because of the unspoken but obvious coercion involved. The very ability of the government to play an effective role in operating or financing a system of charitable response to health care needs relies on its power to coerce cooperation. But this is just the interference with personal liberty that the strict libertarian will not brook.[30]

The difficulties of libertarianism in application are analogous to its theoretical problems. First is the difficulty of maintaining the distinction between negative and positive rights. As already indicated above, libertarianism can accept a great deal of public action and investment in the protection of negative rights. But the more governmental action that is tolerated to provide access to other services, the less compelling becomes the line that should separate legitimate negative rights from illegitimate positive rights. For example, a libertarian society would have to guarantee access to agency investigations, police, and courts in claims about injury due to industrial pollution. Protection of this negative right thus would commit a libertarian government to a great deal of interference, not to mention the taxes needed to raise the public funds necessary to pay for these services. All forms of protection against and compensation for diminished health resulting from the intentional or negligent conduct of others would require similar governmental action and coercive taxation. If this much interference were permitted, why not further action to provide for basic health care outside an exclusively compensatory framework? Clearly, interference itself is not the barrier.

More important perhaps is the problem of the assignment of responsibility for damaging someone else's health, on which the negative right to compensation is based. In a technologically interdependent society such as ours, persons' health may be damaged in countless subtle ways. How does one assign responsibility for ambient air pollution caused by our reliance on the automobile? Yet that reliance was consciously fostered by business and governmental policy. It was government, for example, that elected to build highways instead of mass-transportation systems to American suburbs. Who can avoid the preservatives in the food chain of a society now dependent on highly processed foods, which are inspected and regulated by public authorities and with public funds? Who is responsible for the peculiar stresses of modern life, for the ways we work and play and for the multitude of governmental action already touching on these activities? What share does the public have in the lung-cancer rate, given government subsidies to tobacco growers? As we have seen, diminished health is highly correlated with poverty. To what extent does society as a whole bear responsibility for the poverty amid affluence characteristic of American life and for the deteriorated health conditions associated with it? Surely some of these factors are products of individual choice. But just as surely many of them are determined by broad social forces. If that is so, if society is at least partly to blame for some of the health hazards to which all of us are exposed, then society has a compensatory obligation to those who suffer from the conditions it helped to foster. And since the extent of social responsibility in any given case would be impossible to measure, an appropriate social response might be to ensure a right to basic health care. Such a right would cover whatever social obligation is owed to individuals who suffer and have their lives shortened because of social factors over which they have little or no control. In other words, by expanding the notion of responsibility, even a negative right to health noninterference might be extended to include a compensatory right of access to health care. And it would make a good deal more humane and economic sense to provide preventive and primary care to discharge this social obligation than to wait to compensate the sick, the injured, and the estates of the prematurely dead.

Finally, it may be that the whole emphasis of libertarianism on noninterference, although well meant, is misplaced. The intent of this emphasis is to preserve a range of personal liberty. To do so, prohibitions are placed on the actions of other persons and on government. This is certainly an important moral emphasis in light of the history of political and social tyrannies and especially so in this age of totalitarian statism. But if the goal of libertarianism is to preserve a range of personal liberty, then it must be recognized that forces other than those of persons and governments restrict personal liberty, too. Illness, injury, and premature death through no action of any person or government restrict or terminate personal liberty. The impersonal forces of nature and the only indirectly personal impact of social and economic realities shape and misshape personal liberty every bit as much as, perhaps more than, the direct acts of persons and governments. In light of these realities, the goal of libertarianism might better be captured, not by a ban against interference with personal actions, but by opposition to the domination of rational agency by any forces.[31] Put this way, a society would have to weigh the relative effects of coercive taxation against the coercive impacts of increased pain, suffering, disability, and premature death due to persons' inability to attain access to needed health care. It would then choose the course of action that seemed most likely to liberate the real development of persons' rational agency from all dominating forces. A society committed to this practical approach to personal liberty would not simply rule out a social response to health care needs as a matter of principle.

The second practical difficulty of libertarianism concerns its probable impact on people's lives. Does it make sense to accept a theory of justice that simply dismisses as irrelevant the results of the natural lottery, all considerations of happiness and desert, and even access to the conditions necessary for the development of rational agency. Suppose that a society developed a standard of affluence for most of its members unheralded in history. Suppose that among the minority of the disadvantaged were born an infant needing an operation that the child's parents could not afford, in spite of their very best efforts. Suppose further that the cost of the operation, although prohibitively high for the parents, were not very high, given the average spending in the society on luxury items and recreation. Finally, suppose that with this operation, the child would develop normally, have an average longevity, and become a rational agent. Without the operation, the child would experience considerable pain, have a markedly shortened life expectancy, and be profoundly retarded for all of his or her days. According to libertarianism, it would not be unjust to refuse to provide this child the needed operation because the child would have no right to it. Society might be obliged out of charity to do something for the child, but a pure libertarian society's private efforts might well be ineffective. Although a modified libertarian society might feel obliged to raise public revenue (coercively) for the child's care, it, too, would not have to provide the operation because the nature of the modifed libertarian response is born in freely determined charity, not in a right to have basic needs satisfied. But if a theory of justice, even in its modified form, can have this sort of unpalatable result, how credible is it? Does it not make more sense intuitively to say that this child would have some rights, some claim in justice against its affluent society?

Consider, too, the implication of libertarianism's rejection of desert as a criterion. If two individuals need a heart transplant and only one heart is available, some decision-making procedure must be employed. Under libertarianism, the heart will go to whoever can afford to pay for it. One may assume under a pure libertarianism that if both candidates are able to pay a given price, the price will be bid up until one can pay and the other cannot. Any other alternative restricts these individuals' personal liberty to transfer values. But suppose that one candidate is health conscious and dutiful in diet and exercise, but is the chance victim of another's violence. The second candidate is a lifelong cigarette smoker, a heavy consumer of alcohol, and obese; suppose even that this is a second transplant, the first having been caused by the same factors. None of these desert considerations is morally relevant for libertarianism. And since libertarianism cannot distribute randomly (this violates rational choice) or by the likely result of the operation on each candidate's future life (it eschews result considerations), the heart must go to the second candidate simply because he or she can pay more for it. It requires a very strong theoretical commitment to libertarianism to agree that this is a just resolution.

Finally, how can a theory that places rational agency at its moral center ignore the effect of the natural lottery on the real development of rational agency? To become a person who thinks and chooses autonomously takes more than luck. It takes, among other things, a mind and body within the range of normalcy, broadly understood. Sometimes the natural lottery determines circumstances for persons in which only the interventions of health care can preserve and foster the development of rational agency. At the least, it is ironic—at the most, perhaps contradictory—to so highly value personal liberty that the social action that is often necessary for the real attainment of personal liberty is disallowed.

The third practical problem with libertarianism is its insensitivity to the positive externalities of health care. Society benefits immeasurably from the good health of its citizens. A healthy population is a more productive work force, is better able to provide for national defense, and, one may assume, is better able and more motivated to carry on the general creative work of a civilized culture. Certainly, the opposite is plain. In a circumstance of widespread ill health, the labor, defense, and culture of a society must be compromised. This point was more obvious in the preindustrial age, when nations and whole regions could be devastated by infectious diseases. To the extent that they have had the practical knowledge and abilities to do so, societies have viewed it as part of their duty to the common good to take public measures to prevent such epidemics and to mitigate their effects when they occurred. Today's disease environment makes the impact of health on the common good less evident, but it is nonetheless real.

Thus it is wrong to regard a right to health care as a benefit to individuals but a burden on society. A guarantee of entitlement to some degree of health care can also be a substantial benefit to society as a whole. This point is analogous to what might be said of education. Clearly, the immediate beneficiary of an education is the person whose own rational agency has been enriched and expanded. But just as clearly, a whole society benefits from an educated citizenry in its economic, political, and cultural life. Much of the foundation of contemporary society would be undermined without widespread education among citizens. Similarly, widespread physical and mental health and a reasonably full life span for most citizens is a public good. Libertarianism's inability to acknowledge the common good that results from guaranteed access to health care counts against it.

The fourth difficulty in applying libertarianism involves the original acquisition of health care possessions. If it is fair to regard medical expertise as a possession of health care professionals, as some libertarians do,[32] then the justice of this ownership relies in part on the initial acquisition of medical expertise. If it was not acquired justly, compensation is due. But note that the very posing of this issue in a practical context exposes a deep flaw in libertarianism. How are we to address this question? How can we meaningfully identify the original acquisition of medical expertise? Probably our prehistoric ancestors, even our prehuman ones, knew rudimentary things about stopping the bleeding of wounds, about which foods were healthful and which had medicinal properties, about care for those in childbirth and for the sick and dying. Being unable to determine the relative justice of those first acquisitions, we can assume either that they were all just, thus validating the origins of the status quo in a wholesale fashion, or that the violence and theft that was probably endemic to these early societies affected even those acquisitions, making all the original acquisitions and the entire status quo built on them unjust. Either path seems to result in overly crude moral judgments.

If we focus instead on original acquisitions closer to our own experience—say, the advances in health care made during the past two centuries—another feature becomes obvious. Nearly all these advances required medical research. In addition to the efforts of the medical researcher, such enterprises normally require two other things. First is the heritage of scientific and medical knowledge available to the researcher as a social given. Thus, for example, the most modest contemporary clinician knows more about bacteria than did Louis Pasteur. Of course, this is not so because the genius of modern clinicians matches that of Pasteur, but because the accomplishments of all the world's Pasteurs are now readily available as a collective possession in books, computers, and courses of study.

The second thing necessary today, as it was to Pasteur and to all those who have advanced health care, is the cooperation of nonmedical persons as subjects in medical experiments. Too often, we fix on the efforts of the Pasteurs and fail to see that their accomplishments depended on the use of others. Sometimes these nonmedical others were healthy volunteers; sometimes they were desperately ill and dying "volunteers"; sometimes they were not volunteers in any sense at all. But however they came to be involved, they were the historical co-workers of medical science and clinical application.[33] The acquisition of medical knowledge, then, relied not on an individual combining labor directly with nature, but on the use of individual labor with the crucial public additions of a social fund of knowledge and of countless nonmedical persons as research subjects. And the massive investment of public resources in medical research in the past fifty years or so would also have to be added to these social debts of health care professionals.[34] The conclusion that seems to follow is that those who now possess health care expertise own that expertise unjustly unless some compensation is made. Since the individuals and the heirs of the individuals responsible for these public contributions cannot be identified and compensated personally, an appropriate compensation would be one made back to society generally. The guarantee of an equal right to some basic level of health care for all might be such a compensation. This point is all the more compelling when one considers that historically, the subjects of medical experiments have largely come from among the worst-off—the poor, the sick, those in institutional settings.[35] Since their heirs are likeliest among the worst-off now and would benefit the most from access to basic care, guaranteed entitlement to basic health care might be an appropriate government rectification.[36]

Finally, the transfer of medical expertise as a possession raises practical problems for libertarianism. We know from the Hippocratic Oath that the transfer of the health care skills of physicians in the early but postliterate days of Western medicine occurred within a tightly controlled guild, open not on the basis of personal liberty to exchange values, but on the basis of family connections and social status.[37] This tradition continued into the modern period. Until quite recently, the transfer of physician expertise in the United States wholly excluded women and members of racial minorities. Today's medical profession still bears the marks of a class privilege incompatible with the free rein of rational agency.[38] The organized American medical profession is a tightly controlled monopoly that has historically insisted on protection from the market forces that otherwise follow from a commitment to governmental noninterference in the liberty to exchange values. Although this monopoly has been granted on the basis of the interests of the patients served by physicians, it is also plain that it has served the self-interests of physicians as well.[39] For example, a large measure of control over the number of persons to whom the transfer of physician skills is made in medical schools has been granted to physicians through their accrediting agencies. This public concession was made because of the need to control the quality of medical education, but it also serves to control supply and thus to drive up the prices of physicians' services, helping to make physicians the highest paid professional group in American society. At the same time, this control has helped to make health care harder to find and to afford for many members of the general public. Additionally, much public money has been invested in medical education and in the hospitals that serve both as clinical classrooms and as physicians' work places.[40]

The issue of justice in the transfer of health care resources becomes even more salient in the context of lay-controlled, for-profit provider organizations. Consider this scenario: individual X acquired resources unjustly— say, by defrauding individual Y. These resources were passed to X's heirs. The present holder of these resources, X3, invests them in a major investor-owned, for-profit hospital chain. Suppose that hospitals in this chain refuse care to those who are uninsured and unable to pay. And suppose further, to close the circle, that Y's descendent, Y3, is denied needed ER care at one of X3's hospitals, care that he might have been able to pay for had ancestor Y been able to bequeath his just holdings to him. Admittedly, this is a fanciful sketch, but it shows some of the implications of interpenetration between the general economy and health care provision. In such a circumstance, a historical injustice in the general transfer of holdings would have been introduced directly into the health care context.

All these considerations raise questions about the justice of the transfer of medical expertise and ownership and suggest the need for compensation to society. Since no amount of historical work and subjunctive speculation will allow us to describe a pattern of redistribution that would compensate precisely those who have been treated unjustly by these transfers, an appropriate governmental rectification might take the form of a right to basic health care for all. Again, this would surely aid the least well-off—those who have likely inherited the consequences of these injustices.

Importantly, guaranteeing this right would not necessarily place a direct duty on health care professionals. Instead, the duty would fall on society collectively. Obviously, society does not provide health care; health care professionals do. But society could discharge a duty to ensure access to health care for all by creating social institutions through which individual patients and individual health care professionals could meet in mutually satisfying therapeutic relationships without the coercion of either party. A right to health care does not mean, therefore, the loss of liberty on the part of providers. Just as teachers are free to choose to work for public schools, doctors could make free choices to join publicly operated or funded professional groups, clinics, or hospitals.[41] All these social organizations could be located and structured so as to guarantee access to health care for all. Evidence suggests that even if such a society-wide initiative took the form of a national health service, physicians, because of their unique competences, would remain in an exceptionally strong position with respect to determining the forms of reimbursement for their services and their general working conditions.[42] Thus the suggestion that a social commitment to a right to health care entails the forced labor of health care professionals, although effective hyperbole, does not raise a real moral issue.

Some concluding remarks on libertarianism's claims about envy are appropriate. First, the psychological motivation behind a claim about justice is, strictly speaking, irrelevant to the question of the validity of the claim itself. A law suit, for example, may arise for any number of reasons: envy, hatred, love of justice. But the judge or jury may not decide the case on the basis of considerations of the plaintiff's alleged psychological motivations (which, when unspoken, are largely conjectural), but on the merits of the issue at stake. Similarly, whether or not the claim for greater equality in access to needed health care is an expression of envy is quite beside the point. Second, the fact that greater equality in access to health care and throughout society generally has been urged by many who are among the most fortunate indicates that even if the motive for some who make these claims is envy, envy is not the motive for all.[43] Third, if envy is the pernicious psychological state that libertarianism takes it to be, then it would seem to make sense to try to prevent its occurrence, by condemning not only the psychological state itself, but also the material conditions that give rise to the psychological state. In other words, the surest cure for envy born of extremely unequal circumstances is to make those circumstances more equal. Finally, if a social setting in health care or otherwise breeds widespread envy, there is a self-interested reason why those who have what others envy, and indeed society in general, should strive for more equitable conditions. Uncontrolled envy in the wrong set of circumstances breeds violence.[44] What could be more opposed to the protection of personal liberty, which is at the core of libertarianism, than a society beset with violence. It may seem fanciful to suggest the possibility of the use of violence to secure health care, and perhaps it is when taken out of its social context. But the claim for a right to health care is connected to the general issue of the right to a fair and decent share of the goods and services available in any society. Historically, when other means have proved ineffective, violence has been used to try to attain this goal. Whether the motive is envy or love of justice is irrelevant. When those who are denied turn to violence, everyone's personal liberty is threatened.

Libertarianism, therefore, is a useful reminder of the importance of personal liberty and the need always to justify the actions of the government, but it does not provide an adequate account of justice in theory or as applied to health care. Moreover, reflection on the complexities of libertarianism's demand that government rectify past injustices appears to allow a conceptual opening for securing a right of access to basic health care, an implication that is clearly at odds with the theory's main thrust.

Theodore Lownik Library
Illinois Benedictine College
Lisle, Illinois 60532

6

Contractarianism

An entirely different theory of justice from that of libertarianism emerges if stress is placed on two other implications of viewing persons as rational agents. The first of these emphases is easily seen by attending to the etymology of a synonym for the term "rational agency"—"autonomy." To be a rational agent is to be autonomous, a self-determining individual. An examination of the roots of the word "autonomy," *autos* and *nomos*, reveal two concepts in a curious tension.[1] *Autos* signifies the self, suggesting stress on the individual as the final locus of choice. An autonomous person chooses for himself or for herself. This is the element of free agency in the characterization of an autonomous person as a free and rational agent. But the other root, *nomos*, signifies law, suggesting that free agency is constrained by rules. The autonomous self not only chooses, but chooses in a rule-bound or lawlike fashion. This is the element of rationality in the notion of a free and rational agent. Autonomy requires free personal choice, but it also requires that choice follow some regulation in an intelligent or a rational manner. And this regulation that restricts the self must be freely imposed by the self. Only in this way can a person be both free and rational, both self-directing and intelligent.

The moral point can be expressed in another, more familiar way. This is important, since etymology should not be made to play too great a role in discussions of justice. Usages of words change, and with these changes, meanings are altered as well. But there is greater constancy in human behavior. It seems evident that when personal freedom is used without rules, it tends to destroy itself. Freedom without boundaries becomes irrational and arbitrary. When any action is considered acceptable just because it is freely chosen, freedom leads to irresponsibility. The consequence of this sort of license often is the termination of real freedom in addictions, compulsions, or external limitations imposed by law or by the social judgments of others. Thus the real exercise of freedom requires the constraints of rules and the moral discipline of responsibility. But if these limitations on freedom are imposed on persons by others, individual freedom is lost. Hence the only formula for enjoying real freedom is for the individual to impose regulations on his or her own freedom.

The second element needed to move beyond libertarianism is a frank acknowledgment of our social nature. In order to be free and rational agents in any humanly recognizable fashion, we must be social beings as well. It is paradoxical but probably true that self-confident and mature individuality requires significant childhood socialization.[2] The autonomy made possible by the ability of adults to discipline their own freedom appears to require an earlier disciplining by others. By contrast, a childhood without boundaries imposed by others appears to lead to an adulthood racked with extraordinary and freedom-compromising anxiety.[3] Psychological speculation aside, it certainly seems clear that some persons are born into social circumstances in which their chances to enjoy a reasonably effective range of free choice are lessened or lost from the start. Birth into abject poverty or into a society dominated by violence can make autonomy an unattainable abstraction. In spite of its denial of the relevance for justice of the natural lottery, libertarianism admits this point in part. It insists on the need for government to control violence and threats of violence precisely because in a social environment dominated by violence, real personal freedom is impossible. Thus it admits that freedom is not simply a personal property, but is, at least in part, a social achievement.

But so is rationality. It is plain, for example, that no one becomes rational in private, but requires the social interactions needed to acquire language and logic from others.[4] This point sheds light on the psychological paradox just noted: rules of thought and behavior must be learned from society before a person can become a genuinely autonomous individual. And reliance on social rules is a key ingredient in an individual's rationality. Libertarianism also makes a partial admission of this point by insisting on the government's role in enforcing contracts and prohibiting fraud. The rational structure of an individual's choices relies on the ability to form reasonable expectations of others' conduct, based in part on contracts and on others' representations. But if contracts can be breached and fraudulent representations made with impunity, the social structure of rational expectation of others' conduct is lost. When the rationality of social relations is lost, an individual's ability to make his or her own rational choices is compromised as well. Hence the rational agency of the individual depends in part on the rational structure of the wider society. Personal autonomy requires a social context.

The social contract

A different theory of justice follows from consideration of the significance of persons' free and rational agency when these two points are stressed: autonomous persons must freely bind themselves to rational constraints, and they must do so as social beings. Justice, therefore, can be viewed not as the system that results from the just acquisitions and transfers made by free and rational agents, but as the system that results from the free and rational choices made by persons to impose rules on themselves as a society. Thus justice is a function of the free consent of persons to bind themselves together under rules agreed to by all. Because justice involves a binding agreement among free and rational agents, it is based on a contract. The contract must also be accepted by all, since if agreement is not unanimous, some persons will have rules imposed on them by others without their autonomous consent. The resulting theory of justice is thus a social-contract, or contractarian, theory.[5]

Of course, it is obvious that no such explicit social contract ever existed in any society, nor is it likely to be brought about. There have been historically important social agreements that have helped to shape conceptions of justice in America—the Mayflower Compact and the Constitution, for example. But unanimous agreement among all members of a society on the substantive nature of justice, even in outline, is practically impossible. Consequently, a contractarian view of justice cannot be based on a real social contract, but must appeal to a hypothetical one. Thus justice, according to this position, is to be determined by what free and rational persons would agree to if they were faced with the task of framing a social contract that would command unanimous consent.

More content can be added to this hypothetical situation by recognizing that no such real agreement would be practically possible. What makes it impossible to forge unanimous agreement on even the most basic of social policies in actual societies? The evident explanation lies in the vast inequalities of individual circumstances, the diversity of persons' viewpoints on what is best for society, and the plurality of personal interests. In other words, the rationality of real persons is colored by their unique positions in society. One might say that it is a fact of human nature that one sees justice from one's own perspective, a perspective that must be considered arbitrary, given the accidents of birth into the social environment that shapes that perspective. The slaveholder in eighteenth-century America, for example, was likely to understand slavery through his or her own domination over others, to view the common good as tied to the maintenance of slavery, and to have a whole range of personal interests at stake in the question of the justice of that institution. A person born into slavery at that time, to the extent that his or her rationality was not thoroughly compromised by these social circumstances, saw things from an incompatible perspective. Why each had his or her view probably had more to do with the morally arbitrary fact of birth into a certain race and social position than with any free and rational choices. One need not deny the reality of personal free choice to admit the overwhelming influence of these socially defined perspectives. Given these facts, unanimity on the justice of slavery was not to be expected.

But since the contractarian model is based on a hypothetical contract, the arbitrary differences among persons can be erased theoretically. One can imagine a contract being made, not by real persons, but by hypothetical ones. Such hypothetical contractors can be conceived to be free, rational, and equal. Equality can be achieved by imagining these persons to be placed behind a veil of ignorance, which would effectively deny them the knowledge of the arbitrary facts about themselves and their situations that systematically bias real decision making and prevent unanimity.[6] These contractors can be conceived to be ignorant about their race, gender, age, strength, or intelligence in the real society. They can be denied even the knowledge of their own conception of the greatest good, ignorant about whether they have a religious world view, for example, or, if so, which it might be. Contractors can be imagined to know only the most general facts about human nature: that persons and societies differ in their situations and views on life, that different things motivate different persons, that there are a variety of talents and abilities, and so on.

It follows necessarily that in such a situation, rational agents could not know their specific interests. Hence the task of constructing the rules for justice in society would have to be cast in the very broadest terms. Contractors could not concern themselves with crafting rules for the distribution of goods that they as individuals created or desired to possess, since this would be unknown. Instead, they would have to design principles for the distribution of goods that depended on their cooperative social interaction and that every human could be presumed to want. Therefore, their attention would center on the primary social goods of liberty, opportunity, wealth, and self-respect. They would be interested in principles for the distribution of these primary social goods because these general goods facilitate access to all other specific goods. If the contractors were also denied any altruistic concerns for one another in general, they would not be concerned about the distribution of goods on the basis of charity, but only about distribution following strictly from justice. Contractors behind this sort of veil of ignorance can be thought of as free, rational, equal, and mutually disinterested.

But they would also be self-interested. Whatever principles of justice they agreed to behind the veil of ignorance would be the general rules that they must eventually live under.

The grounds for contractarianism can now be stated more precisely. Justice in a society is defined by the basic principles for distributing primary social goods that would be adopted unanimously by free and rational persons behind a veil of ignorance, which would render them equal and mutually disinterested. Although this hypothetical construct is complex, the moral point at issue is simple. One *should* choose morally the way one *would* choose rationally under conditions that made bias impossible. Or put in other terms, one *should* do in real circumstances what one *would* do in ideal circumstances. Contractarianism can be thought of as a way of imaginatively freeing our better selves from the real circumstances that too often cause us to become arbitrary in our choices. These are the realities that incline us to favor our own interests and further our own conceptions of what is best in prejudice to the different interests and conceptions of others. The device of a veil of ignorance is meant to shut out the knowledge that makes bias and self-serving choices possible and inevitable. If the basic principles that would be adopted unanimously for society by unbiased contractors can be determined, then these principles should be used as standards in our real society. Since these principles define the distribution of access to the primary social goods, they are the bases on which we can say that persons ought to have rights to these goods. Thus the exploration of a hypothetical contract gives the basic principles of justice, which, in turn, generate a framework for articulating the rights that persons ought to have.

What would contractors behind a veil of ignorance choose as the basic principles for society? Each would be unaware of any specific needs, but each would know that he or she had needs. It would be rational, therefore, for each contractor to try to maximize his or her individual share of the primary social goods. This strategy would ensure that whatever his or her particular needs, each would have the best possible general goods with which to try to secure them. Each contractor would weigh proposed principles from this point of view: What will this pattern of distribution of this primary good mean for my chances to enjoy a full range of specific goods in a real society? This consideration would create a powerful inclination toward equality of shares, since no one would want to risk having a significantly lesser share. Like the cake cutter who must take the last piece after all other pieces have been chosen, contractors would have a direct personal stake in creating equal shares. Each would know that he or she might get the last and, therefore, least share.

Each contractor would also know that persons have natural differences and that their situations vary. This fact may necessitate some inequalities. If, for example, only 1 percent of the population has the requisite skills for a necessary but difficult job—say, the mathematical design of computer pro- grams—the good of society may require the use of special incentives to call out and reward that talent. Multiplied across all society's jobs, this use of incentives in the face of varying work interests and capacities may generate considerable social and economic inequalities. Knowing that this is likely, contractors would select social principles that ensure that even the minimum share of the primary social goods would be the best share possible. As rational agents, each would agree to maximize the minimum share of primary social goods because each would know that that minimum share might really be his or her own share. Sometimes this would entail agreement on equal shares; sometimes, on the largest minimum shares.[7]

Specifically, it can be assumed that hypothetical contractors would insist first on a principle guaranteeing the greatest amount of personal liberty compatible with an equal amount of liberty for everyone else.[8] As free and rational agents, they would value liberty highly and understand that it is a prerequisite for the enjoyment of most other goods. Moreover, they would insist on equality. Not knowing, for example, if he or she will be slave or free, each would reject slavery. Unaware of individual race, each would reject racism. Denied knowledge of gender, each would reject sexism. This pattern of reasoning would prevail until all forms of differential personal liberties were rejected. Thus the personal privileges that these systems allow for the slaveholder and for the dominating race or sex would be rejected because these personal privileges for some mean domination for others. None of the contractors would risk being among those others, but would insist on equality for all. Some other restrictions on liberty might also be acceptable, might even be mandatory, if they were imposed equally and served to extend liberty overall. Traffic lights, for example, impede imme- diate liberty of movement, but extend liberty in general because they make travel by car relatively safe. These sorts of restrictions would be acceptable. But the basic principle would be to distribute the greatest amount of equal liberty possible. This first agreement would provide contractors with a principle of justice that gives rise to a wide range of negative rights of noninterference.

Next in importance to liberty is opportunity. But since opportunity is shaped so directly by wealth, contractors would have to decide on a princi- ple for the general distribution of wealth before considering principles to govern opportunity.

They would know, let us assume, that societies differ in terms of the overall wealth that is available for distribution. Some societies are rich; some, poor. Suppose that they also know that one of the ingredients needed for creating wealth for distribution is the efficient use of a society's natural and human resources. To achieve this efficiency in light of persons' differences in talents and productive capacities, incentives are sometimes useful. The employment of such incentives can cause social and economic inequality by, for example, raising the income of some relative to that of others. Thus in order to maximize a society's wealth so that all may benefit, it may be necessary to allow some to benefit more than others. But the justification of this differential in income must make reference to the benefits that this arrangement conveys to all, especially the least advantaged, persons in society. Otherwise, there would be no reason for the contractors to agree to differential incomes, knowing that each of them might be the one with the smallest income in society. But there would be a reason to agree if even the smallest income were made larger than otherwise possible by the wealth generated by the higher income of others. Thus for the distribution of wealth and income, contractors would agree to a difference principle: differences in wealth and income are acceptable, but only so far as they serve to maximize the wealth and income of the least advantaged persons in society.[9] This principle allows the generation of positive rights of access to the wealth of society within the constraints of allowing for socially useful differences.

Contractors would then be concerned to ensure that the jobs and offices to which differential incomes were attached were open to all. They certainly would not accept the possibility of being arbitrarily excluded from seeking higher-paying jobs for themselves. Equality of opportunity in seeking jobs and offices would therefore be part of the social contract. And because they would know that the natural lottery can tend to arbitrarily exclude persons at their very starting points, contractors would insist on a social guarantee of compensatory measures that tend to mitigate the impact of the natural lottery. Public education would be guaranteed in order to mitigate the arbitrariness of being born, for example, into a family of illiterates, since such a starting point may foreclose the opportunity to compete for jobs and offices fairly. Thus the equality of opportunity that contractors would agree to is not only an in-principle openness of all jobs and offices to everyone, but also a social guarantee of measures that make the actual operation of equal opportunity as fair as possible for everyone.[10] This principle forms the basis for a range of positive rights of access to those goods and services that, like remedial education, serve to make pure competition for jobs and offices also fair competition.

Contractors behind a veil of ignorance who sought to reach unanimity on the selection of principles for the just distribution of primary social goods would therefore agree to three principles. In the distribution of liberty, they would agree to the greatest possible liberty compatible with an equal amount of liberty for all. In the distribution of offices and jobs, they would agree to fair equality of opportunity. In the distribution of wealth, they would allow differences in income, but only to the extent that these differences worked to the benefit of the least advantaged person in society. These, then, are the three principles that should be applied to a real society. What free, rational, equal, and mutually disinterested persons would agree to as just is what real persons should employ as the standard of justice.

There is one additional primary social good—self-respect. It is primary because it is a condition for the real enjoyment of most other goods. It is social because social conditions can dramatically enhance or diminish the chances of any individual achieving it. Its just distribution is served by the use of the principles of liberty, opportunity, and wealth, since each person thus is respected by others as an equal and incalculably worthy individual and is guaranteed the social framework necessary for self-respect. But one further stipulation is called for. The preservation of a just distribution of self-respect requires that the three principles be satisfied in order of priority: liberty, opportunity, and wealth. This means that liberty cannot be exchanged for greater opportunity, or liberty or opportunity exchanged for greater wealth. It would be demeaning to the self-respect of persons and subversive to social relationships among equals to allow the bartering of fundamental personal liberties or opportunities in exchange for enhanced income. Selling oneself into slavery or trading away one's vote, for example, are acts of disrespect to the self. To have this done by others, even for greater personal income, is a fundamental injustice. Free and rational contractors would not allow such trading. They would insist on equal liberty and fair opportunity and would permit differences in income only so far as they served the least well-off; and they would insist on the ordered priority of liberty, opportunity, and wealth to ensure persons' self-respect.[11]

If contractarianism were applied to the issue of employee rights to health care benefits, the nature of the benefits would first have to be established. Are they a primary social good in the society under consideration? This question must be asked first, since the social-contract approach is not meant to solve all distribution questions, but only those of the most basic sort. Put another way, contractors are to fashion principles governing just institutions, which then generate their own rules. From these principles and rules, persons' rights will follow.[12] Let us assume that in this society, health care benefits were a primary social good because they were an important form of wealth. The benefits would have to be distributed either equally or, if incentives are appropriate, on the basis of maximizing the position of the worst-off employee. The application of the difference principle might come into play if the use of benefits as incentives could generate more resources for benefits overall. Then inequality of distribution would be just, if the employee receiving the smallest benefits still got more as a result of this arrangement than he or she would receive by a more strictly equal distribution. These factors would have to be appraised from a contractor's point of view—that is, on the assumption that each contractor might be the least well-off employee. Unanimity would be made possible only if that position is the best it can be.

Assuming that liberty is not an issue in this case, one other question of justice remains. Presumably, the employer would have the job of determining the amount and distribution of employee health care benefits. The employer, then, not only would have access to a primary social good in wealth, but also would hold a special job or office. Opportunity to hold this job must be open to all equally and fairly. If the job required special skills—say, managerial or accounting training—then fairness would demand that the employees have access to the means, perhaps education, of attaining these skills. This would ensure that the job of employer were fairly and equally open to all, even if at a future date. The employees would have a right to this sort of practical access to the jobs of their society, and they could not accept greater health care benefits in exchange for their fair equal opportunity to become employers. This would violate the proper ordering of the principles of justice and undermine the foundations of the employees' self-respect.

Contractarianism is an important perspective on justice. Its emphasis on the social character of freedom and reason is an important corrective to overly individualistic theories. Its model of contractors framing the basic principles for institutional justice provides a useful thought experiment, a way of detaching oneself from the press of immediate claims about justice and rights in order to gain a wider point of view on the very purpose of cooperation in society. And the specific principles generated are both historically significant and rich in contemporary application. Nevertheless, contractarianism, too, can be charged with major theoretical difficulties.

First, it might be objected that the very hypothetical structure of social-contract reasoning leads to practical irrelevance.[13] That no such contract ever did or ever will exist in fact is an important reminder of the ideality of this system. How useful is it, then, in criticism of the real world? Specifically, does it not make more sense intuitively to begin with actual historical persons, define their rights on the basis of realities about them, and then fashion just social institutions around these rights? But contractarianism begins with a hypothetical situation, from which it derives principles for a just society and only then the rights of persons. Is this not an inversion of the natural order of reasoning? Moreover, what kind of persons are these hypothetical contractors? By being situated behind a veil of ignorance, these alleged individuals lose everything on which individuality might be attributed: race, gender, national identity, social position, strengths and weaknesses, even a personal sense of the ultimate goods in life.[14] Although rational, the contractors also appear to be exceptionally cautious. Would not some real people prefer taking a risk on being in the privileged position in an unequal society, if the stakes were high enough, rather than demanding that the worst situation be the best it can be? In more general terms, the contractarian view uses the veil of ignorance to build in an equality among persons at the very outset.[15] But this is one of the most controverted issues in real societies and real debates about justice: Just how equally should persons and their conceptions of life be considered? Finally under the charge of unreality, is it appropriate to regard the natural lottery as morally unfair, as something for which social compensation is due?[16] Again, the circumstances determined by the natural lottery are facts; the work of the contractors is ideal.

Second, the problem with compensating for the natural lottery can be located specifically at the principle of fair equal opportunity. Given that simple equal opportunity to secure jobs and offices is insufficient to overcome inequalities in starting position, how far must a society go in correcting natural inequalities in order to make competition for these jobs truly fair?[17] Must everyone be provided with remedial mathematics education, for example, until there are no mathematicians more able than others for jobs requiring mathematical skill and to which differential income may be attached? What of the personal charisma apparently necessary for political leadership? Must remedial personality courses be available until everyone is equally able to run for president in terms of personal charm? More seriously, how far must society go to remedy or compensate for severe mental and physical disabilities? These and similar problems abound once there is a principled commitment to substantively fair equal opportunity.

Third, when using the difference principle for distributing wealth, how are the least well-off to be identified?[18] In the distribution of health care benefits, the answer is easy: the person with the fewest benefits. But given the complexities of the forms of wealth in society and the equally complex dimensions of human needs and desires, how shall we know the truly worst-off? Surely, abject poverty is a first obvious indicator, but where does one look after this: the victims of racial and ethnic discrimination, the educationally or culturally deprived, the sick and the aged, the well-off but deeply unsatisfied? Unless the least well-off can be described precisely, the standard for justifying the redistribution of wealth will be unclear. Furthermore, in real societies, redistribution of the possibly radical sort called for by contractarianism would require taking from some people what they now own. From the libertarian perspective, this is itself unjust.[19] But the application of the difference principle, although redistributive, might still leave vast inequalities, justified by the role they play in making the worst-off better than under any available alternative. This raises questions of justice from the egalitarian perspective.[20] And there is no guarantee, because there is no conceptual linkage, that contractarianism would tend to maximize overall happiness in society by distributing wealth on the basis of the difference principle. One can assume that contractors would not be interested in the overall happiness in their society, only in ensuring the largest minimum share of primary social goods for themselves.[21]

Finally, one can challenge the ordering of contractarianism's principles. Maximizing the minimum condition would not of itself guarantee that the minimum condition would provide a humanly decent standard of living.[22] The best that the minimum share can be might not be good enough. Imagine a developing society in which persons would die of starvation unless they allowed talented others exclusive liberties to amass personal wealth. With these privileged freedoms, the fortunate few would be able to create, in the process of seeking their own benefit, just enough social wealth to avoid mass starvation. Would it be unjust or a subversion of self-respect for the near-starving masses to agree to such an inequality in personal liberties, if by doing so starvation could be avoided and greater economic security could be had for all? Put simply, is it never right for a society to trade freedom for bread, not even if want of bread threatens to make freedom an illusion for the great majority? Contractarianism's ordering of principles seems to rule out such trades, but it seems that, as tragic a choice as this might be, a trade of freedom for bread might sometimes be the lesser of two evils.

There are, of course, contractarian responses to these objections. The theory is purposely ideal because the real world is never fully just, and it must be criticized from an alternative and unbiased point of view. Persons' rights do not simply follow from their natures but evolve through social institutions, some of which are more, some less, just. Therefore, knowledge of the principles that make for just social institutions is needed to uncover persons' rights. Real persons, of course, are not behind a veil of ignorance, but this is precisely what makes them so often impervious to moral considerations. They are tenaciously and unconsciously committed to their own interests, as defined by their natural and social positions. The presumption of equality among the contractors is a mechanism to ensure an intuitively fair process of reaching an agreement. Any other assumption would build in biases that would make unanimity and, therefore, the autonomous self-imposition of rules impossible to conceive. Real persons' willingness to take risks is generally conditioned by their desire to overcome the unsatisfying real circumstances they are in. Contractors would not be driven to risks because the character of their social circumstances would be under the control of their unanimous agreement. And the natural lottery must be considered unfair because it is arbitrary. No one deserves his or her parents or the natural and social conditions at the start of their lives.

Fair equal opportunity is a principle whose application in specific societies would have to be made by means of a democratic political process. Clearly, fairness cannot guarantee strictly equal opportunities because the natural lottery disadvantages some beyond the means of any society to repair. What it does mean would be contextually determined by the nature of the jobs and offices available, the relative affluence of the society, and the kinds of disadvantages that persons face. A general theory of justice cannot be expected to determine fairness in particular circumstances.

The specific norms for the use of the difference principle would also require democratic choice. In an open political process, those allegedly least well-off would make their case for that status, and the majority would have to decide the merits of the various claims made. Clearly, deprivation of life's basic necessities is among the most compelling cases that the allegedly worst-off can make, since all other people are subject to the same needs. Redistribution would be required by the difference principle; in the social-contract view, this does not violate the ownership rights of those who have an unjustly large share of wealth. Rights are not prior to, but follow from, the principles of just distribution. Inequalities would likely remain, but, again, they are acceptable if they make the worst lot in life better than it would otherwise be. These inequalities follow from the factual differences among persons that no theory of justice can erase and that no efficient society can afford to ignore. Of course, utility might not be maximized in a contractarian society. But no individual contractor would be rationally concerned about the net amount of happiness, only the share that he or she may draw.[23]

Finally, contractarianism can allow that it may sometimes be true that the trade of freedom for bread may be the lesser of two evils. But when it is, such a choice follows from the exigencies of catastrophe or near catastrophe, not from considerations of justice. Justice as a virtue of social institutions operates only in the great space between a surfeit, such that everyone has all they need, and a deprivation, such that social cooperation is impossible.[24] It operates in the context of relative scarcity. When a whole society is in the condition of absolute or near-absolute scarcity, considerations of justice are suspended in favor of what needs to be done for survival. In such dire circumstances, the choice to trade freedom for bread may be necessary. If so, this is lamentable, but not unjust. Justice simply has no application in such extreme circumstances.

Contractarianism, therefore, provides a plausible theory of justice. It generates three ordered principles applicable to all social institutions: maximum equal liberty, fair equal opportunity, and inequality of wealth as long as it benefits the least well-off. Use of these principles in a real society will give rise to three corresponding human rights: a wide range of noninterference with personal freedom, access to goods and services that foster fairness in the competition for offices and jobs equally open to all, and a share of society's wealth as large as is needed to justify the greater wealth of others.

Liberty, opportunity, and wealth

How would contractors behind a veil of ignorance approach the question of the right to health care? Each, of course, would be denied knowledge of his or her own health status. Thus the contractors would not know which of them had been born prematurely or with genetic defects, which needed a great deal of pediatric or geriatric care, which would ever be pregnant, which would suffer from debilitating accidents or chronic illnesses, which would have impaired cognitive abilities or other psychological handicaps, or which would suffer and die from what diseases and under what conditions. The contractors would know, let us assume, that all these conditions prevail in their society and that each contractor is at risk. Assume further that they know that unless specific agreements are made to the contrary, it may turn out that some of the real persons with these needs would not have ready access to health care.

It would be rational for contractors to take steps to see that health care would be readily available to address all these needs. Each would be motivated to ensure the best possible minimum share in life, and since each might have the need in question, he or she would want to be sure that the best appropriate health care is available even to the persons worst off in society. This much seems clear. The more difficult question is to determine under which of the three principles for just institutions health care would fall. This is an important question because its answer will help to confirm the intuitive sense that contractors would agree to guaranteed access to health care. Even more important, locating health care under one of the three principles will provide a better idea of the scope of the right to health care that alternative institutional arrangements may generate.

If the right to health care is located under the equal-liberty principle, the first implication is the creation of a contractarian right of health noninterference. But contractors might go further and regard good health as being as fundamentally important as liberty itself.[25] Serious compromise of health certainly does compromise one's exercise of other liberties. In the extreme case, death denies an agent all natural liberty. Physical and mental impairments may cause the loss of real liberty to travel freely and to choose for oneself. Lesser medical conditions may not seem as directly related to liberty, and many of the trivial ills of life probably are not. But even some of the lesser conditions may have a negative impact on personal liberty if they are not treated early and properly. As far as health care is efficacious in preserving a degree of health conducive to the exercise of liberty, health care becomes instrumentally related to the most important primary social good. By implication, then, basic and effective health care may itself be considered an important primary social good, second only to the liberty it facilitates.

If health care is a primary social good on the order of liberty, then its distribution would be governed by the first principle of justice. Each person would have a right to the widest possible range of health care compatible with an equal amount of health care for all. Thus on this account, contractarianism demands an egalitarian right to health care, one probably best expressed through a public system that would ensure equality of access.[26]

Obviously, it would make no rational sense to distribute care in a way that is mechanically equal to all, but unresponsive to differing individual circumstances. This would not be a rational contractor's goal. Instead, equality of access in this context would be based on need, since this is the concern that would motivate the contractors' agreement. Since they would be committed to equality in matters bearing on liberty, contractors would agree that similar needs warrant similar treatment regardless of ability to pay. And they would insist on the greatest amount of equal care possible. But the greatest possible may sometimes be none. It is possible, one might suppose probable, that under this scheme, all persons with diseases that are very expensive to treat would not be treated, or that those few who are treated would be selected by a method—by lot, for example—that respected their equal moral rights.

Additionally, since liberty itself can be restricted in some circumstances as long as the restriction is equal and serves to secure a greater share of liberty for all, the same would be true for health care. It might be desirable, for example, to cease aggressive treatment of any person regardless of disease condition when the prognosis for further success reached a certain degree of unlikelihood.[27] Health care resources saved by restraint in these marginal cases could then be used to satisfy other health care needs. Just as liberty can be restricted at stop signs to secure greater liberty on the roads for all, so health care expenditures could be limited to allow for greater health care investment elsewhere, as long as everyone in the same situation were treated in the same way. What would be disallowed, given the priority of the principle of justice, however, would be any trade of health care resources for opportunity resources or for wealth. As a primary social good on a par with liberty, health care could be traded for more health care, but not for any lesser goods.

Most of the strengths and weaknesses pertaining to an egalitarian basis for a right to health care apply to the contractarian view of health care as liberty. Its major strengths are the primacy given to a right to health care and the self-respect that a system of guaranteed equal access for equal need would engender in society. Its main weaknesses lie in the economic costs that such a system would likely entail and in the limitations on the freedom to purchase additional health care that a unitary system might require. The irony of the last point is that some liberty might itself be compromised when health care is valued as highly as liberty. Liberty can be traded for greater liberty, and therefore health care for greater health care. But can liberty be traded for greater health care and vice versa? Since the pure theory of contractarianism places liberty alone in this first position and since the argument for placing health care there too is its value in preserving and enhancing liberty, the application of the theory to the distribution of health care may require an ordering within the first principle itself. This would mean that health care could be traded for greater liberty, but not liberty for greater health care. With this amendment of the contractarian view, a sacrifice of some of the value of an exclusive unitary system would be necessary to allow for the liberty to purchase some services outside the system. But this exception could not be taken too far before the basic right to the greatest possible health care compatible with the equal right of others would be lost.

The second contractarian approach locates the right to health care under the second principle, fair equal opportunity.[28] In order for persons to compete fairly for equally open jobs and offices, they must have equal life opportunities in the very broadest sense. This might be defined roughly by reference to the normal functioning typical of a member of the species, at least as that expresses itself in the society at hand.[29] In other words, a broadly equal life opportunity means the ability to formulate and pursue the life plans typical of normal persons in one's own society.

Since poor health can compromise the ability to function normally and since this can mean the loss of fair equal opportunity to pursue the offices and jobs available in principle to all in a just society, health status is an important variable in determining real opportunity. To the extent that health care is effective in preventing, curing, or compensating for health-related conditions that diminish opportunity, health care would be a right.[30] Its distribution would be based on need, and it would be distributed equally with respect to need; but health care need itself would be judged in the light of its impact on opportunity. In other words, the goal of guaranteeing a right of access to health care under this version of contractarianism would be to maintain, restore, or replace normal functioning.

The virtue of such clarity on the goals of health care is twofold. First, it helps to avoid the problem of conflating desires with needs.[31] In this account, health care needs relate to what is necessary to ensure normal functioning. Health care desires do not relate directly to ensuring normal functioning, but to enhancing states of health that are already normal.

Satisfaction of the needs is a right; satisfaction of the desires is not. For example, access to plastic surgery needed to restore normal function of a burned face would be a right, but access to plastic surgery to remove the effects of normal aging would not be a right. Second, tying the right to health care to opportunity blocks a potentially endless demand for the commitment of health care resources in cases—terminal illness, for example—where the attainment of normal opportunity even in its broadest sense is not a practical possibility.[32] This does not imply that health care would not be provided to the dying and to others in hopeless conditions. Health care can be provided on bases other than that of persons' having a right to it. It may be provided out of compassion or a sense of decency, for example. In these cases, providing whatever health care is appropriate is not a matter of the just arrangement of social institutions, but of charity.[33]

An opportunity-based right to health care would have the same status as a right to public education.[34] Like education, health care would be publicly distributed to guarantee the attainment of a minimum degree of functional normalcy so that the conditions of competition for offices and jobs would be broadly fair. Some persons would require only a standard amount of health care to attain the normal range, as they require a standard educational curriculum. Others would require considerably more care of a remedial nature. Still others would be in conditions in which health care services were incapable of reaching the goals of normalcy and provision of care, and these cases would fall outside what is mandated by justice. Assimilating health care to the model of education also reveals the reasonableness of focusing available resources. Most of our educational resources are concentrated on the young, since youth is the time of life of greatest need. Contractors can be presumed to know this. They would also know the statistics relating to health care needs and would agree to focus on them, always with an eye toward achieving maximum normalcy for those who are capable of attaining it. Thus as education is focused on the young, so health care might be focused on the old, on young children, or on the unborn.[35]

Another consequence of placing health care in the same category as education is that competition for opportunity-related social expenditures is thereby revealed. Investment in health care would have to be weighed against investment in education and in other areas, such as housing, employment, and general economic development, that have a known impact on fair equal opportunity.[36] It is likely that the basic kinds of health care— ordinary perinatal and pediatric care, emergency care, and primary care, for example—would prove to be every bit as important as basic education in securing the functioning typical for individuals in a given society. Thus this kind of care would be guaranteed as a right in any just and reasonably affluent society. But more expensive and less demonstrably effective health care—heart–by-pass surgery and some organ transplants, for example—would have to be judged in comparison with the incremental advance in preserved or restored normalcy that a similar investment in education or job-training programs might make. If the weight fell on education, the right would lie there and not with more health care. Rights to health care or education in this context are thus not direct, but are derivative from the right to fair equal opportunity. In preliterate societies and in the early history of medicine, neither education nor health care was meaningfully related to the attainment of normal ranges of opportunity. Thus there was no right to either, although there was still a right to fair equal opportunity. These observations make clear the dynamic and society-specific character of derivative rights in an opportunity-centered contractarian theory. To the extent that the efforts of social institutions are effective in achieving normalcy for persons relative to other possible efforts, persons have a right to these social efforts. But the primary social good to which there is a right is fair equal opportunity, not health care itself.

The likeliest institutional arrangement for the recognition of a right to health care in a contractarian society with an opportunity-based distribution principle is a two-tiered system. The first tier would provide socially guaranteed health care tied to the goal of preserving, restoring, or replacing the level of functioning considered normal for persons in that society.[37] The ability to pay would be irrelevant in this tier because of this care's direct connection to the right of fair equal opportunity. The range of health care provided in this tier would be determined by a social judgment as to its efficacy in securing normal opportunity compared with that of other possible uses of the resources invested. The second tier would be a system in which persons would be free to purchase any additional health care goods and services, whether or not they related to opportunity. Thus the first tier would establish a right to a minimum amount of health care, up to that needed to achieve normalcy. The second tier would be a free market for health care in which there would be no positive rights of access.

The third contractarian alternative locates the right to health care under the difference principle.[38] Health care goods and services are considered a form of wealth. Since contractors would be concerned to maximize their minimum states, the distribution of this wealth would be presumed equal unless the least well-off could be made better off by an unequal distribution. Because wealth can take so many forms, describing how health care would be distributed as a form of wealth in a contractarian society is inherently complex. Three general simplifying strategies are available. First, health care can be considered a form of wealth separated and closed off from other forms. In this closed case, the difference principle is applied directly to the distribution of health care. While contractors would certainly be rationally motivated to apply the difference principle to all forms of wealth to ensure the largest minimum share for themselves, the closed distribution scheme supposes them to regard health care as important enough to be treated separately. The second alternative is a wholly open model, in which health care is considered one form of wealth among many. It is accorded no special separate status. The difference principle is applied to wealth as such, and the implications for the distribution of health care are derived from the general pattern of wealth that results. The third alternative has elements of both the other systems. This mixed view regards health care as special enough to deserve some separate treatment, but not so special as to be closed completely to influence from the general pattern of wealth distribution.

In a closed system, the application of the difference principle would lead to the equal distribution of health care based on need unless an unequal distribution would improve the condition of the least well-off in terms of health status. This might entail large inequalities. The very sick would plainly be candidates for more care than others on grounds of need. Therefore, this closed system of wealth-based contractarianism would mean large investments in health care for the very sick, regardless of their prognoses for recovery. Indeed, the more negative the prognosis, the worse off the patient; the worse off the patient, the greater the justification for more health care—except, perhaps, if it would confer little or no benefit. Contractors can also be presumed to know that some illnesses can be prevented or lessened by preventive measures. They might therefore regard pregnant women, fetuses, and young children as populations of greatest need for preventive health care. This would require an understanding of the meaning of "worst off" in terms of potential—that is, worst off unless a preventive intervention occurs. This definition may seem awkward conceptually, but would not be difficult for contractors to apply because their entire task of framing principles of justice would involve making choices among possible societies. The balance between investment in treatment and investment in prevention would have to be struck in a way that respected their fundamental interest in ensuring the best possible minimum state in a closed health care–distribution setting. Whatever the balance, the best delivery mode would probably be a public health care system for all. Persons would have a right to the health care provided by this system when they fell into one of the categories of need that was covered.

Distributing health care in an open setting would have different implications. In this system, health care resources are considered to be simply one other form of wealth, a form interchangeable with others. The easiest method of distribution in this setting would be to apply the difference principle to income generally and not to health care itself. Thus income would be distributed equally unless an unequal distribution would make the income of those with the lowest income higher than it would be under a pattern of equality. Individuals could then decide for themselves how much of their own general income to invest in health care and whether to do so on an as-needed basis or through investment in insurance. Income differential would be available to stimulate the production of needed goods and services, including those related to health care. For example, income incentives to construct hospitals, to develop new drugs, or to train for the health care professions would create inequalities of wealth in society. If access to these goods and services made even the least well-off economically better off because of increased income directly or because of enhanced productivity due to better health, then the difference principle would be satisfied. This strategy would likely be best effected through the encouragement of a plurality of delivery systems, perhaps in a free market. A significant feature of this approach is that there is no right to health care as such, but only a right to a certain level of income. And it also follows that just as persons would be free to invest that income in any way they chose, they would be free not to invest any of it in health care.

The third general strategy for a wealth-based contractarian distribution of health care would be a mix of features from both the closed and the open systems. In this setting, the difference principle would be applied directly to health care in order to establish a public system for the distribution of health care based on equal treatment for the needs that the society could afford to cover. Extra investment would still be mandated for those with the greatest health care needs. At the same time, the difference principle would also be applied to the general distribution of income, permitting the consequent inequalities that would benefit the least well-off economically. But since this approach does not regard health care as wholly closed to the rest of the economy, additional purchases of health care beyond those covered by the public system would be permitted. Thus, for example, if the public system could not afford to make artificial hearts available to all who needed them, those who could afford to pay would be allowed to purchase them outside the public system. This would result in an ultimately unequal distribution of health care beyond that which would be socially guaranteed, but contractors might agree to this if the general pattern of income distribution were fair. The result would be a right to a fair minimum of health care, a right to an income justified by the difference principle, and the freedom to exchange some income for additional health care.

In summary, there are three contractarian approaches to the right to health care, corresponding to the three principles of justice. A liberty-based conception gives rise to an equal right to health noninterference and, if health is taken to be as central as liberty itself, to the widest possible range of health care possible for all. This care would be provided, most likely, through one public delivery system. An opportunity-based conception allows a right to the health care necessary to attain the level of functioning normal for a typical person in a given society when such a level is attainable. Charity would provide the basis for the care of those too ill to approximate normal functioning, and a second tier of care would be permitted for the purchase of care beyond normalcy for those who can afford it. Finally, a wealth-based conception can apply the difference principle in three ways. One would give rise to a public system with an equal right to needed care, except if the very sick or those at high risk to become very sick could benefit from more care, to which they would then have a right. A second would guarantee a right to only a difference-principle-justified income, and health care could be purchased with that income in a multitude of ways. A third would provide a right to needed and covered health care in a public system, a right to a difference-principle-justified income, and the ability to satisfy uncovered needs and desires outside the public system with personal income.

Of course, there are objections to the health care applications of contractarianism. Some of them mirror the theoretical problems described earlier, and some are more specific to its implication for the distribution of health care. Of global significance is the rejection in principle of hypothetical reasoning and of the whole construct of free and rational contractors. Because of its theoretically general nature, this objection can be passed over. In application, contractarianism either is or is not useful in determining the outlines of justice in health care delivery. The proof of this is not in theoretical argument, but in appraisal of the fruitfulness of the application itself. Arguments specific to health care application are of greater concern now.

The right to health noninterference of the liberty-based conception is an important, but a very limited negative right, as we have already seen. The stronger view that there is a positive right to the greatest equal amount of health care may be criticized on its first premise—that health care is so essential to liberty that it is to be ranked with it as the most fundamental of primary social goods. As important as the instrumental connection between liberty and health care is, the connection remains just that—instrumental. The categorical difference between the two goods becomes plain in a moment when one considers history. Persons and nations have fought and died for their ideas of liberty. Surely nothing of similar import can be said of health or health care. Even if it is admitted that the effectiveness, and hence the value, of health care has increased dramatically in the past several decades, it still seems almost absurd to think that persons and nations would fight and die for health care. Second, many other social goods are instrumentally necessary for the exercise of liberty. Lack of food, clothing, and shelter can impair or destroy liberty, too. But as important as this makes these goods, we would probably not suppose that justice demands that they be distributed on the basis of the greatest possible amount compatible with an equal amount for all.

Third, in spite of problems with the distinction, it is broadly true that liberty is a negative right of noninterference, but a claim to health care is a claim of a positive right of access. Noninterference rights are theoretically satisfied by everyone's nonaction. This is why one can so readily speak of an equal right to the broadest possible liberty. Aside from the practicalities of police protection, courts, and the like, these rights are relatively easy to guarantee and relatively free from conflict with themselves. A right to the greatest amount of health care possible with an equal amount for all, however, might require a public outlay of substantial resources, resources taken from private individuals. This at least raises the question of the abridgement of others' liberties. So, too, does the potential need to curtail access to care by any when similar care cannot be had by all. But these possibilities for interference with liberty suggest that a principle combining liberty and health care distribution may be in conflict with itself.

A contractarian position based on opportunity has the potential for limiting public commitment to health care to a more manageable size. But even on the basis of this account, there will be some individuals—those who need organ transplants, for example—who may be capable of attaining normalcy, but only at massive social costs. Moreover, realizing the savings possible by limiting the right to health care to a normal chance for fair equal opportunity is possible only so far as what is normal and what is fair are clearly made out. What is normal functioning in a society is itself partly shaped by the level of health care available to its citizens. There may, therefore, be a circularity in defining access to health care by reference to normal functioning. Additionally, persons may have any number of serious health care needs that do not impair their normal functioning; high blood pressure and the early stages of cancer and heart disease are examples. Would they have no right to care until normalcy was lost? In terms of fairness, just how far must society go in using health care to even out the natural lottery? Would a person with an unsightly nose, for example, be considered at an unfair disadvantage in job interviews; if so, would plastic surgery be a right following from fair equal opportunity? Finally, there is a certain counterintuitive quality to the implication of the opportunity account for those who are incapable of attaining normal functioning. The very persons one might expect to have the strongest claim for a right to health care—the very sick, the dying, those who are so far from normalcy that they cannot care for themselves at all—are excluded from a guarantee of entitlement to care.[39] Instead, they must rely on charity, an all-too-often undependable source of health care.

The problems of the wealth-based account of contractarianism stem from the difficulties of defining the least well-off and of framing the proper relationship of health care to the general economy. If the worst-off are defined in terms of health care needs and the health care system is closed to the rest of the economy, an egalitarian need-based system emerges. Besides the expense and the other problems typical of such a system, the fact that this system is closed allows the possibility that even those who were made relatively wealthy by the general application of the difference principle will have their health care paid for publicly. If the system is open, the needs of some, determined by the natural lottery, may overwhelm their income, while others, quite arbitrarily, have considerably lesser needs. The possibility also arises that persons will not anticipate their own health care needs accurately, but will exhaust their otherwise fair income on other goods and services. One might be inclined to say that this is a consequence of their own free choices, but health care needs are literally unpredictable. Denying care to those who cannot pay will not be made much easier by the knowledge that given other choices and under other circumstances, the needed care might have been afforded. There is also the difficulty of justice to the health care needs of children and other dependents of persons who have exhausted their fair incomes elsewhere. A mixed system of closed and open elements mitigates the worst problems of each, but is also subject to the problems of each. Are the worst-off the sick or the poor or the sick poor? Would the presence of nonpublic alternatives lead to too much inequality? Would they tend to drain resources away from the public system? And the whole wealth-based approach of every version is conditioned by the priority of the other two principles. Whatever rights may be derived from these accounts are qualified by the priority of liberty- and opportunity-related rights.

Contractarians, of course, can respond to these challenges. Health care may not be the same as liberty, but they may be so closely associated by the effectiveness of modern health care that denial of access to the first amounts in practice to inability to exercise the second. Just as one liberty can be exchanged for another, so health care can be exchanged for liberty and vice versa. And it may well be that a principle of the greatest equal amount of all the basic necessities of life would be agreed to by contractors as directly demanded by the liberty principle. Surely, contractors would have no rational interest in abstract liberties that they could not exercise for want of minimum satisfaction of life's basic needs. Guaranteeing a right to health care may be costly, but it is a social cost that must be borne in justice if the contractarian scheme is to be broadly valid.

An opportunity-based distribution scheme would indeed depend on clear definitions of the concepts of normalcy and fairness, but they cannot be defined abstractly without context. Each real society must define them and redefine them as conditions change. Principles can act only as guidelines; they cannot of themselves determine specific policies. There is a circularity in normalcy's interdependence with health care, but that is to be expected. A society's standard of normal functioning is a product of all the interactions of natural and social factors. And duties of charity are not by their nature any more subject to failure than are duties of justice. Societies can fail on each count and be equally condemned for both. The strength of the opportunity account is in its delineation of the appropriate application of each kind of duty.

The application of the difference principle to health care as a form of wealth is certainly a complex matter. The determination of the least well-off person in a democratic society would issue from a political process to which every citizen would have fair and equal access. It is not clear that contractors would be bound to regard the delivery of health care as either closed or open on principle, so this decision, too, might be left to the prudence of a real society's democratic deliberations. And a right to health care based on the difference principle is preceded in importance by rights to liberty and to opportunity, but it is unlikely that just health care delivery would conflict with these other rights, fairly interpreted.[40]

Many of these objections and replies arise from the question of where to locate conceptually the delivery of health care in a society governed by the principles of a just social contract. But as important as these particular controversies are for a final appraisal of contractarianism, they should not be allowed to obscure the wider thrust of this theory of justice. Would free, rational, equal, and mutually disinterested persons faced with the task of framing the principles for a just society agree unanimously to guarantee entitlement to some degree of health care? Would persons behind a veil of ignorance who were trying to secure for themselves the best possible minimum condition insist on a right to health care? Assuming that they knew the efficacy of modern health care and the consequences for their liberty, opportunity, wealth, and self-respect of being unable to obtain health care, it seems that the answer to these questions would be yes.

7

Plural Foundations

Three of the theories of justice we have considered—utilitarianism, egalitarianism, and contractarianism—allow for a straightforward articulation and defense of a claim to a right to health care. Although the general thrust of libertarianism opposes this claim, emphasis on the social factors that affect individuals' health characteristics and on the social debts incurred in the acquisition and transfer of medical knowledge and skills provides a plausible compensatory basis for recognizing a right to health care. Thus all four theories of justice might be used to validate a claim to a right to health care. Is the case for a right to health care therefore proved? And which of these theories provides the most complete proof? Which provides the correct account of justice on which the case for a right to health care is properly based? Responses to these questions require an examination of the nature of proof as it might be used in this context.

Proof and persons

There is a political sense in which the claim to a right to health care needs proof in the United States. Because no such general right has been recognized legally in the United States, the burden of proof falls on those who would argue that it is incumbent on government to guarantee entitlement to some degree of health care for all its citizens. That burden is lessened somewhat by certain other political facts: international agreements that the United States has signed declare health care to be a right; every other industrialized democracy effectively recognizes such a right by providing or financing some level of care for all its citizens; and acceptance of this right is consonant with certain existing elements in the political culture of the United States—specifically, the national commitment to Medicare and Medicaid.[1] Nonetheless, since the status quo acknowledges no general right to health care, proponents of the right must bear the burden of proving the case politically. In this instance, having the burden of proof means having the responsibility of marshaling the necessary popular consensus in an open political process.

One obvious reason for resistance to the claim to a right to health care is the cost that such a right might entail. But although important, this consideration is not compelling in itself. Historically, no positive health care right was recognized when costs were not so high. Even in the present situation of costly health care, spending limits could be set by establishing fair rationing policies. An affluent society can certainly afford some level of basic care for all its citizens. A deeper reason for resisting a right to health care is to be found in the individualism characteristic of American traditions.[2] One dimension of this individualism is a political disposition to distrust government. But as powerful as this inclination generally is, it has been overridden in contexts where it became plain that personal and local initiatives, even under the best of circumstances, were insufficient to the enormity of the national task at hand; the New Deal is a case in point. Of course, even if Americans did decide that providing universal access to health care ought to be a national priority, interest-group politics would shape or even deflect a national response.[3] These are realities that any attempt at political reform must confront.

There is a more specific explanation for resistance to a right to health care in the United States, and that explanation lies in the very legal framework of society. American common law is exceptionally individualistic. This feature is most plain in the tort-law doctrine that defines the duties of persons to come to the aid of another who is in peril of injury or death. Except in the case of family members, the common law recognizes no duty to aid another person unless the would-be rescuer has done something to freely assume that responsibility.[4] Even if a person in need will die without assistance and another can provide that assistance at little or no risk, that other is not legally liable for having refused to render the needed assistance. This means, for example, that an adult who observes an unrelated child drowning in a swimming pool is not legally bound to do anything to help the child. Even if this adult is a superb swimmer, he or she is not required under law to swim to the rescue, to throw a handy rope, or even to shout for the assistance of others who are less unmoved by the child's plight. The point of this morally shocking legal doctrine is the presumption that the law should hold an individual to obligations only when they arise out of the responsibilities of family roles or are freely taken on by the agent. The mere juxtaposition of one person's need with another's ability to aid does not constitute a legal requirement to render aid because the social relationship of one person to another is thought to be less compelling than the individuality of each. In the area of health care, this doctrine has been used to justify claims that physicians and private hospitals have the right to refuse treatment to medically needy persons even in cases of emergency.[5]

Among industrial democracies, the United States stands alone on this legal doctrine, at least in its application to health care.[6] Even Great Britain, from which the United States inherited the doctrine, has avoided its health care implications by establishing the National Health Service. And the main reason why other nations have taken a different road on this legal duty to aid is clear. Although many factors must be considered in judging the advisability of putting a moral intuition into law,[7] no moral theory could justify the outrageously callous behavior of an adult who is observing a drowning child and is not attempting some form of rescue.

This moral insight provides a different perspective on the burden of proof involved in claiming a right to health care. The situation of someone in dire need of health care can be likened to that of the drowning child; indeed, there are causes of death that precisely mimic drowning (pneumonia) and medical rescues that are little more difficult than throwing a rope into a pool (injection of penicillin). Despite the law in the United States, there seems to be a consensus that a drowning child has a valid moral claim on a nearby adult for lifesaving assistance. If this is so, then by parity of reasoning, the same child dying of pneumonia should have the right to an injection of penicillin. If a child may also claim the right to be assisted so as not to fall into a pool in which he or she may drown, then the same child should also have the right to the care needed to avoid pneumonia. And the analogy can be widened to encompass social responsibility. If ten adults were at the side of a pool, a drowning child should have the right to be aided by at least one of them. Better yet, if children are known to have drowned in the pool, children have a right individually and the adults have a duty collectively to see that a lifeguard is always present when children are swimming. Then to the extent that health care is merely a specific form of aiding those in need, would it not appear to follow that society ought to recognize a moral right to some basic level of health care, a right of access to a medical lifeguard?

The point of this simplifying analogy is to show that the claim to a right to basic forms of health care ultimately has the same moral standing as the claim to a right to be rescued. It seems intuitively evident that persons have a moral right to be rescued when they can be and where no great risk is entailed for the rescuer. In these circumstances, the rescuer has a moral duty to render aid to those in need. But what could be said if someone demanded that this most basic moral intuition be proved? Certainly, each of the theories we have examined could provide some grounds for a response, but each has its own presumptions, which might be challenged as well. Compared with the abstract considerations presented by each of these theories, here is a more rudimentary and concrete issue: Can it be proved that society or anyone is responsible to answer the claims of a person needing rescue? Can a moral duty to aid be proved?

At this most fundamental level of morality, the question of the burden of proof becomes of crucial significance. Must those who recognize the moral obligation to aid others in need prove their position? Not necessarily. The duty to provide aid to other persons in need may be such a basic premise that from a moral perspective, it is virtually self-evident.[8] If so, the burden of proof lies with those who would deny any duty to aid. William James may have put this best. He held that "without a claim actually made by some concrete person, there is no obligation, but that there is some obligation wherever there is a claim." In the face of a claim or a demand for aid, the burden of proof is reversed, falling not on those who assert a right to the aid but on those who deny it. "Take any demand," continued James, "however slight, that any creature, however weak, may make. Ought it not, for its own sake, to be satisfied. If not, prove why not." The only such proof that James thought morally possible would appeal to the existence of incompatible obligations to other persons. Only other moral obligations can stand in the way of acknowledging a moral duty to aid, and not the amoral or immoral presumption that there simply is no obligation to aid others in need. At this most basic level of morality, the obligation to respond to the needs of others is, according to James, simply a matter of "life answering to life."[9] Practically, the moral imperative to aid those in need is a presumption that morality must make. Cognitively, it is an act of knowing that cannot be derived from anything more basic; hence, it is a primary moral intuition.

This is not an abandonment of reasoning, but a recognition of reasoning's proper role in morality. Morality, it must be remembered, concerns practical matters, the norms that shape human conduct. Reasoning in morality therefore must arise from and return to the arena of human conduct. That arena is itself conditioned by certain broad realities about human existence. Fundamental among these existential realities is the fact that persons rely on the help of other persons. This is not an incidental fact about people, but one that is universal and essential. From our prolonged helplessness in infancy and youth to our constant reliance on the multiple others who nourish, educate, and provide all the goods and services necessary for human life, we stand in need of other persons. Morality cannot be oblivious or neutral to this fact. Instead, it must presume the goodness, rightness, and, in general, obligatory character of aiding those in need. Thus a general moral imperative to aid those in need is not a conclusion to be reached by moral reasoning, but is a presumption it must start from—a practical, existential presumption.

From a cognitive point of view, that one should come to the aid of another person in need must count as the most basic of moral knowledge. Indeed, one may think of it as closely related to the prescription of the golden rule—to take the other's point of view. One may think of the mandate to come to another's aid as a specification of the general golden rule command of reciprocity to the case of need. Or one may just as easily regard the golden rule itself as a generalization to all human relationships of what is morally obvious in the face of human need—that a necessitous other must be helped.

If the obligation to aid those in need thus requires no special moral justification, the derivative claim that there is an obligation to provide health care to those in need may require no elaborate justification either. It is simply an application to a specific group of persons with a specific set of needs of the moral intuition of a general duty to aid those in need. To move from this point, that a claim of health care needs entails an obligation to aid, to the recognition of a social duty to provide health care based on the rights of persons to receive it, is thus not so large a conceptual step. Certainly, the burden of establishing a right to health care given the existence of a prior obligation to aid those with health care needs is not that of proof. Instead, it involves the lesser burden of creating a reasonable case that rights and duties are the proper ways to interpret the obligations at hand. In other words, the existence of a right to health care does not have to be proved, but only shown to be a reasonable implication of the duty to aid those in need in health-related contexts. The difference might be captured by appeal to the different standards of proof applicable in criminal and in civil law. In criminal law, the standard of evidence is tantamount to proof: beyond any reasonable doubt. In civil law, the standard is less rigorous and amounts to only the making of the better case: preponderance of evidence. Similarly, if a moral right to health care has to stand on its own, it has to be proved in such a fashion that no reasonable person could doubt it. If, however, it can rest on the more general and virtually self-evident moral intuition that there is an obligation to aid those in need, then the establishment of a moral right to health care requires making only a reasonably persuasive case. Part of the importance of this point is obvious. Reversing the burden of proof on the existence of a duty to aid and then resting the case for a right to health care on this presumptive duty makes it far easier to argue for a right to health care. A good part of the case for a right to health care is already carried by simply applying the prior moral duty to aid to the context of health care needs.

But there is a second advantage to this position that is important, too. This approach to the right to health care not only makes a difference regarding the relative strength of the argument needed, but also affects the kind of argument needed. If the moral basis of the right had to be proved, it would probably require a continuous line of reasoning built on one or a small set of accepted premises. To secure the conclusion against all reasonable doubt, a deductive or nearly deductive method based on a definitive theory of justice would be necessary. For example, a contractarian might have to show that only the social-contract approach to justice is valid and that given this approach, a clear line of demonstrative reasoning leads from the most general presumptions about the conditions of agreement on a social contract to a right to health care. Were such an argument made, it would be exceptionally strong from a logical point of view. But it would have two highly vulnerable points. Both the plausibility of competing theories of justice and any failure to demonstrate entailment of a right to health care from the social contract would give rise to reasonable doubts.

If, by contrast, the case for a right to health care does not require proof but only a persuasive case, then it is not necessary to rest it on only one theory of justice and on a deductive inference of a right to health care from that theory. If the ultimate basis of the right is not a theoretical claim about the nature of justice, but a morally obvious practical intuition about the duty to aid those in need, a pluralistic approach is possible. The case for a right to health care can then be built on several theories. Utilitarianism, egalitarianism, libertarianism, and contractarianism can be used as four ways to articulate the more rudimentary intuition that there are obligations to those in need. These theories arise because of the need to express and defend varying interpretations of the demands of justice. Justice is morally necessary in society because of the scarcity of goods to be distributed. Practically, therefore, the concern for justice begins with the fact of persons in need. Hence, the several theories of justice can be viewed as various ways to specify the practical moral intuition that there is a duty to aid those in need or, at least, to provide an explanation of the other moral obligations that preclude such a duty. Understood in this fashion, insights and arguments from each theory can be used as long as they are not mutually contradictory. And generally, the main feature of these theories that threatens to make them incompatible is the implicitly exclusive character of each. But this feature can be removed simply by making the modest assumption that no one of them contains the complete account of the demands of justice, but that each illuminates certain key features of this inherently complex human notion. Then we need be wary only that specific arguments developed from each view do not contradict one another. If these arguments do not contradict one another on specifics and do reinforce one another in conclusion, a plural foundation for a right to health care is produced. This foundation will not be logically simple, but it will have persuasive strength.

And it will avoid the vulnerability of resting on one system of justice and one line of reasoning.

There are two additional reasons for adopting a pluralistic approach. One is the sheer variety of the kinds of goods and services important to persons. From clothing and real estate, to lifeguards and social workers, to affection and job satisfaction, human experience is filled with objects, services, and intangibles that persons need and desire. Articulating and defending principles for the morally proper means of distributing all these disparate things is the province of a theory of justice. But the very plurality of things to be distributed argues for a plurality of principles of distribution and even a plurality of conceptions of justice itself. It is simply implausible to assume that some single conception of justice is rich and flexible enough to provide guidance in all these areas. More likely, the things themselves and the circumstances of human need and desire for them will have to inform a useful theory of justice. But if these things and circumstances are many, so, too, must be the theories of their just distribution.[10]

This point is evident when applied to health care. Among the many goods to be distributed are artificial hearts, cadaveric livers for transplantation, dialysis machines, prosthetic devices, hospital beds, X-ray and radiation machines, vaccines, and drugs and medical supplies of all kinds. Services include intensive and coronary care, well-baby check-ups, psychiatric counseling, dental care, home health visits, nursing-home care, genetic counseling, surgery, pathology and other lab reports, and the time and attention of physicians, nurses, and pharmacists. Intangibles that are distributed include physical and mental health, trust and protection of confidence, privacy, professional standards of quality, accuracy and fairness in billing, humane treatment conditions, liberty, enhancement of self-respect, and human concern and commitment. Furthermore, considerations of desert, fairness to providers and taxpayers, and relationship to the larger web of personal and social values must be taken into account. Is it likely that all these things can be properly distributed by one principle or even by several principles derived from one conception of justice?

The final reason for adopting a pluralistic approach is related to the bases on which the several theories of justice are themselves developed. Each may be thought of as resting, more or less, on a certain insight into the nature of what it is to be human. From these different perspectives on the nature of persons, different interests are put forward as morally central to justice. For the utilitarian, people are goal-oriented and sensate beings. Because of this, they have interests in securing satisfaction, happiness, and pleasure and in avoiding frustration, unhappiness, and pain. For the egalitarian, persons are intrinsically and incalculably worthy beings who are deserving of equal respect. Because of this, they have interests in securing the widest range of equality possible in society, since this will best respect the equal value of all persons. For the libertarian, persons are rational agents. Because of this, they have interests in protecting their liberties against the use of force or deception by others. Of all the theories considered, it is least clear that contractarianism presumes a conception about persons because so much of what is real about persons is stripped from them when they are placed behind the hypothetical veil of ignorance. Nevertheless, it is instructive to consider the human features that contractors still have. Contractors are rational, social, and self-interested. Because of this, they have fundamental interests in securing freedom to make their own choices, a range of social opportunities, and the best possible real circumstances for themselves.

When these theories of justice are seen to rely on differing conceptions of the person, the question of which theory is the true or the best account of justice must be refocused. The question now is: Which perspective on the nature of persons is true or the best? Are persons goal oriented or incalculably worthy; are they rational agents or social and self-interested? To ask these questions is to realize that what it is to be human is not simply a matter of fact to be discovered. Clearly, matters of fact are relevant, but comparative judgment of these views puts forward a question of value. Is it more revealing, more fruitful, more in line with other important values to regard persons this way instead of that? These theories are thus as creative as they are factual. This is not to denigrate the important project of speculation about the nature of the person. The point is to see what these speculations really do. On the one hand, like science, they explore realities about persons. But on the other hand, like art, they creatively highlight, compare, and interpret a reality far too complex to allow for definitive factual description.

If these theories do have at least something of a creative dimension, then the question of which theory is true is without clear application.[11] One theory may be better than another in some respects and for some purposes, but for the traditionally persuasive theories considered here, it is not meaningful to ask which is the definitive perspective on persons. There is simply no way to definitively determine the nature of persons or, at the very least, no way to know that any given perspective on that nature is the definitive one. Since the various theories of justice considered here are grounded in an interpretation of persons' nature, no one of these theories can be known to be definitive of justice. Each may be inventive and insightful in its own way. Each may lead to important additional perspectives and comparisons. Each may afford a critical distance on our current beliefs and practices. But none is, or can be known to be, the one true theory.

It follows, then, that if no one of these theories is true to the complete exclusion of the truths contained in the other views, no choice among them is necessary theoretically. As long as the specifics are not contradictory, insights and arguments can be drawn from all the theories. It needs to be added, of course, that not all theories are equally insightful, and some are no doubt factually flawed, absurd, or repulsive to other important values. But this is not the case with utilitarianism, egalitarianism, libertarianism, and contractarianism. They have been considered here precisely because they have long and influential histories, and they command the commitment of many able thinkers today. But with the qualifications that not all theories are equal and that few are as important as the four at hand, a pluralistic account of justice and the right to health care can be produced employing elements from each of the four.

This is not an eclecticism for its own sake. There are specific strengths and weaknesses of each of these theories, as has been indicated. A plural account seeks to include the strengths that can be consistently held together and to avoid the weaknesses. At a deeper theoretical level, this sort of pluralism follows from a certain metaphysical skepticism, a doubt that the most fundamental questions concerning the nature of the person are capable of rational resolution. Such speculations are then regarded, not as competing and incompatible alternatives, but as differing perspectives on an ambiguous and overdetermined reality. Each perspective offers a standpoint from which other interpretations can be derived and other meanings focused more sharply. Developing a concept of justice on this understanding of speculations about the person is therefore not a foundational project, not a project building on a theory that alleges to mirror human nature itself. Instead, it is a conversational project in which several voices, reasoned and persuasive voices, enrich and expand one another's contribution to an ongoing dialogue.[12]

In sum, a pluralistic account of the right to health care recommends itself on the basis of three considerations. If it is admitted that there is a general duty to aid others in need, then the moral case for a right to health care does not have to be proved, but only made reasonable. This can be done without developing one line of argument from one theory of justice. It can be done by employing many arguments and various theories of justice. Second, the multiplicity of goods, services, and intangibles to be distributed in society, in general, and in health care, in particular, makes it likely that more than one conception of justice will be necessary. Third, each of the theories of justice under consideration relies on a conception of what it is to be a person. But these alternative conceptions of the nature of persons include creative elements that are not appropriately judged true or false. Instead, each brings important insights and alternative ways of regarding persons. Therefore, an adequate account of justice and the right to health care will have to take insights from each of these major and influential theories. The conclusion of these three considerations is pluralistic in substance and method. The case for a right to health care can be best made by drawing the most important insights and arguments from utilitarianism, egalitarianism, libertarianism, and contractarianism. And there is one more virtue of a pluralistic approach: disparate strands of argument provide enhanced rhetorical strength. The single view may be thought of as a chain—only as strong as its weakest link. The plural view, by contrast, is like a cable—as strong as the number of intertwined and mutually supporting threads.

Beginning with the assumption that there is a general moral duty to render aid, there are, then, four moral arguments for interpreting this obligation as a right to health care. First, establishing a right would likely increase the average chance of living a long life well and would thus tend to maximize overall utility in terms of persons' pleasure, happiness, and satisfaction. Second, a social guarantee of entitlement to health care would express respect for the intrinsic, incalculably great, and therefore equal worth of all persons. Third, recognizing a right to health care is a just compensation for society's negative effects on persons' health and for social debts accumulated in the acquisition and transfer of wealth, in general, and of health care resources, in particular. Finally, establishing a right to health care is morally incumbent on us because it is part of a reasonable social contract, part of what wholly unbiased persons would agree to as a framework for a just society. Together, these four arguments, drawn from four theories of justice, provide the pluralistic foundations for a moral right to health care.

The nature of this right can be detailed by attending to a problem with contractarianism that may require modification of the theory. If it is possible, and it seems to be so conceptually, that the least well-off persons in society could still fall below a decent minimum condition as a result of the application of the difference principle, contractors might modify their agreement by adding another principle, ordered after the liberty principle but before the opportunity and difference principles. This principle would assert a right of access to a decent minimum share of the necessities of life. It clearly would not be in the interest of any contractor to agree to the difference principle if the least well-off person, although made better off by income differences, could still be below a decent minimum condition of life with respect to access to life's necessities. Furthermore, since the principle of fair equal opportunity is meant to apply to offices and jobs to which income differentials are attached, it should be preceded in importance by a principle of minimum security that would guarantee access to a minimum of life's fundamental necessities.[13]

With this modification, the framework of contractarianism can be used to articulate a pluralistic right to health care based on the four principles of contract theory, but with strong influences from the other three theories.

The right to health care, according to this account, can be viewed as the core element of a bundle of four specific rights.[14] Locating specific rights to specific kinds of health care at each principle allows for the establishment of a priority ordering. The principle of equal greatest liberty would be first and would serve as the basis for a negative right of health noninterference, such as that compatible with libertarianism and procedural egalitarianism. The principle of minimum security would follow, providing the foundation for a universal right of access to a decent minimum amount of health care, including basic primary and preventive care, emergency care, and whatever other kinds of elementary health care a society considers both minimally necessary and affordable for all. This is a broadly egalitarian principle, but with the support of hypothetical contractors' likely insistence on it. The principle of fair equal opportunity would then ground a right to those health care interventions designed specifically to sustain and restore normal functioning when that is possible: surgery in cases with strong positive prognoses, rehabilitative techniques known to restore patients to normalcy, and curative medicine generally. Again, this is what contractors would likely agree to; but it also would allow a utilitarian calculus of health care efforts centered on the attainment of normalcy. Finally, the difference principle would govern the general distribution of remaining wealth. Since a general structure of health care justice would be guaranteed by the three prior rights, the difference principle could be applied in an open health care setting, allowing those with more disposable income to purchase additional forms of health care to satisfy uncovered needs and desires and to buy amenities. The openness of this approach would allow for a range of inequalities that could be organized to promote maximization of utility. And it would permit a large range for personal choices, consistent with the spirit of libertarianism. Of course, providing additional details about the sort of care that would fit under each of the four principles would be a matter of continual adjustment in the contexts of a democratic political process, the changing power of health care, and the general wealth of society.

Several important implications follow when the right to health care is interpreted in this fashion. Placing the right of equal liberty first would protect self-respect because it rules out at the start wrongful violations or diminutions of any person's health, even if great benefits could thereby be attained for others. It would, for example, provide grounds on which to make medical experimentation with human subjects illegal unless the subjects were unquestionably volunteers. The second level of right would guarantee universal access to primary health care, including access by those who cannot be returned to normalcy. Placing this positive health care right prior to any right to normalcy-related curative care would emphasize the moral priority of caring over curing. Most important, it would avoid the counter-intuitive result of denying a right to health care to those who might need it most, simply because they were beyond hope of a return to normalcy. With the possible exception of some forms of emergency care, this right would include access to kinds of health care that are highly personal and less technology intensive. The problem of expense would therefore not be as difficult an issue as it is with high-technology curative health care. In fact, guaranteeing this level of right might actually lower cost overall by empha-sizing prevention, by ensuring prompt entry into the health care system, and by providing less intensive and more appropriate care for the dying and severely ill. Distribution would follow substantive equality, guaranteeing access on the basis of need. This right would probably require governmental action to operate or finance a health care system guaranteeing broad equal-ity of treatment in conditions conducive to the development of persons' self-respect.

The third part of the right would guarantee entitlement to curative and rehabilitative care when the attainment of normalcy is possible. Because of the obvious expense entailed by such a right, it would have to be subject to two qualifications. First, the standard of maintaining or restoring normalcy would have to be used in a rigorous utilitarian fashion, so that only health care of assured effectiveness were used and only in cases where the prognosis for normalcy were very positive. Even with this proviso, care might have to be limited, since claims for resources in health care must compete with those in other areas related to achieving fair equal opportunity. If care must be limited, the principle of procedural equality would have to be observed. Again, the best use of that egalitarian principle would be no treatment for those in certain categories of illness or selection by lottery of those to be treated. Mechanisms reflecting desert, such as taxes on dangerous products or enhanced co-payments and deductibles, could be used here too, not to deny needed care, but to help defer the cost of treating those suffering from their voluntary choices to assume higher health risks. Recognizing rights at this level might require governmental action, but might also be compatible with a mixed public and private delivery system. Such a system would allow for the widest range of experimentation both with health care itself and with methods of cost containment.

The last element of a pluralistic right to health care would preserve the liberty of those with additional disposable income to purchase uncovered and desired health care, including amenities not provided publicly, outside the public system in an open free-market setting. This liberty would defeat a strict egalitarianism, but given the egalitarian elements built into the prior health care rights, it should be acceptable. For the utilitarian, it would allow for the creation of social incentives that might promote maximum happiness, such as experimentation with different health care delivery systems. And for the libertarian, it would provide one clear locus for the free transfer of justly acquired wealth and thus limit the control of government.

This conception of a pluralistic foundation for a bundle of rights built around the core of a right to health care is clearly most compatible with a modified form of contractarianism. But it also clearly shares a great deal with egalitarianism. It describes a system of health care that would discharge whatever compensation is due, on the libertarian account, for society's health care–related debts. And for the utilitarian, this interpretation of the right to health care is based on meeting human needs in such a way that would certainly increase and possibly maximize average utility. It would do so in a way likely to lead to long lives lived well for most persons and, by placing the less costly caring and preventive functions of health care ahead of the curing ones, might help to do so at the lowest possible cost to society.

Rights, charity, and ideals

One last perspective must be considered before the discussion of the right to health care is complete. This view is that there is no positive right to health care, even if there may be an obligation on the part of health care professionals or society to provide it. This position must be examined, since the claim to a right to health care ultimately rests on a corresponding duty to aid. If a meaningful duty to provide health care can be derived from the general duty to aid without appeal to persons' rights, then there is a serious challenge to the conclusion that a right to health care is the most plausible interpretation of the duty to aid applied to health care contexts. From this position, it is not the specific arguments for a right to health care that are flawed. Rather, it is the very starting point of using the language of rights to capture the moral obligations at hand that is rejected. This nonrights alternative may be arrived at in three ways. First, it may be objected that the very language of rights is misleading in general or as applied to health care. Second, it may be charged that the obligation to provide health care arises wholly out of concerns of charity, which give rise to no corresponding rights on the part of the recipients of health care. Finally, it may be held that the decision to provide health care publicly arises neither from persons' rights nor from obligations of charity, but from free choices to be guided by historically evolved social ideals of decency. Social action on the basis of these ideals may generate legal rights, but with no equivalent moral rights.

The first nonrights position rejects the very language of rights. It may be expressed as a general or specific rejection. At the general level, it can be claimed that the concept of a right in its modern usage is a moral innovation. There appears to have been no equivalent term in the ancient or medieval world in spite of the great number of historically important discussions of morality extant from those periods.[15] If Aristotle, for example, could offer such penetrating and perennial wisdom on morality without recourse to a Greek equivalent to the modern word "right," the term may itself be unnecessary or misleading. Even after the term evolved and gained currency, some thinkers rejected it on the grounds that it made moral discourse unnecessarily absolute and thereby produced irreconcilable conflicts. Some have viewed it as placing such an extreme emphasis on individuality as to lead to antisocial consequences.[16]

In the health care context, the language of rights has been rejected for being too adversarial.[17] According to this view, the doctor–patient relationship is founded on the basis of a moral covenant that requires doctors to assume special obligations to patients and to society. This covenantal obligation includes all the protections that others want to provide with the language of rights. In additon, it contains an element of gift that leads doctors to supererogatory efforts on behalf of patients and society. The language of rights, by contrast, leads to contentiousness, litigation, and the practice of defensive medicine. It debases the doctor–patient relationship by changing the personal bond from covenant to contract.

The second nonrights position holds that health care is properly distributed not on the basis of right, but on the basis of charity.[18] The duties required by charity are considered to be as compelling and as important as those required by justice. And they have an additional advantage. Whereas considerations of justice tend to be cognitive and calculating, concerns of charity tend to be emotive and spontaneous. Since health care at its most fundamental is a human response to the sufferings of other persons, the more elemental and existential basis for response is the appropriate one. The very notion of care itself recalls the intimacy of familial relationships in which love, not justice, conditions persons' responses. This charitable concern can be expressed either by voluntary giving or by enforced coordinated effort. But in either case, the moral obligation is on the part of those who provide or finance the care. There are no moral rights on the part of those who receive it.

The final nonrights approach is based on a conception of social ideals of decency. These ideals have arisen and evolved historically and have many sources, including religion, morality, politics, and culture. They constitute a society's living traditions and shape both persons' senses of obligation and their expectations of one another. In modern American society, concern to provide access to health care for all is part of the evolved cultural fabric of obligations and expectations. Just as in another time and place, the notion of socially guaranteed universal access to health care might have sounded impossible or absurd, it strikes many contemporary Americans as plausible, perhaps even morally mandatory. That persons should suffer and die for want of health care in the midst of the affluence of the United States is shocking to this historically evolved public conscience.[19] But there is no strict moral obligation in justice or in charity that demands a response to the need for health care. Instead, commitment to the social ideal of being or creating a certain kind of society is a free political choice made in light of traditional values. Thus a system to guarantee a legal right of access to care can, perhaps should, be established, but there is no equivalent moral right.[20]

These nonrights positions derive in part from a larger view of the nature of human communities. Persons and their relationships are shaped profoundly by the organic character of their communities. In these communities, conflicts must be resolved by careful attention to all the interests at stake and with subtle compromising and balancing. Compared with this social perspective, the language of rights presents a preemptive claim of privilege, an arrogant refusal to acknowledge one's internal relatedness to others and to the community as a whole. Human communities also care for their members out of genuine affection and love. Compared with this natural bond of feeling, the insistence on justice imposes artificial rational regulations that subvert spontaneous concern. And human communities develop and react on the basis of living traditions that sum up their historical experience and give meaning and direction to their present efforts and hopes for the future. Compared with this cultural perspective, the artifice of pseudo-persons making imaginary contracts for societies that never were or will be is an empty exercise detached from moral reality.

These are powerful objections to the entire project of describing and justifying a right to health care, the more so because they recognize to varying extents a duty to provide some level of health care. But there are also compelling responses to these challenges. First, although the concept of a right may not have a clear equivalent in the ancient and medieval worlds, this fact may be a sign of moral progress. Ancient and medieval societies recognized legal slavery, too. Certainly, the fact that Aristotle and virtually all the great moralists of these periods found slavery an acceptable institution suggests that their moral horizons lacked a feature that modern theories tend to have—stress on the central moral value of each person.[21] Furthermore, there are anticipations of the notion of a right in the ancient Stoic philosophy, and all the intellectual background necessary for it is in the medieval concept of natural law.[22] Allowing a place for guaranteed entitlements is a challenge for morality, but rights need not be conceived as absolute. The specifics of an unbundled right to health care would be relative to many factors, including the nature of persons' needs, the power of health care, and the affluence of society. And when rights are put in priority order by a series of principles, conflicts among them are minimized.

That rights introduce a potentially adversarial dimension into the doctor–patient relationship cannot be denied. The very point of the concept of a right is to create an exceptionally strong vehicle for expressing an individual's moral demands. As such, rights are important protections for persons. If persons are worthy of respect as incalculably valuable beings, then some things are wrong to do to them and some goods and services are wrong to deny them. Thus any human relationship has a potentially adversarial dimension as long as persons may be abused in it. There is no good reason to exempt the arena of health care from the respect owed to persons in all relationships. No doubt, the doctor–patient relationship has historically embodied strong covenantal elements, but associated with this achievement have been instances of unjustified paternalism, neglect, and harm to patients. Moral and legal rights are instruments to protect persons from these abuses. The traditional ethos of the medical profession, as important a moral achievement as it is, is simply insufficient to the task. Furthermore, that ethos is under extraordinary economic pressure at present, making appeals to covenant seem more nostalgic than practical.

Charity is insufficient as well. The history of publicly funded or operated health care efforts is the history of the failure of private charity, since if charity had been effective, public efforts would not have been necessary. It is arguable whether "charity" enforced by the state for the purpose of coordinating an effort large and effective enough to address the social need is really charity. To be forced to give seems directly opposed to the voluntary and spontaneous features usually associated with charity. Even if coerced giving were considered a genuine form of charity, it would not necessarily match the needs at hand, since the final standard of giving arises from the discretion of the givers, not the needs of the recipient. And even if coerced giving were somehow to match the need for care, it would still be morally defective. The dependence of the recipient on the charity of the donor is directly subversive of self-respect.[23] Even if the goal of the donor is laudable and the need of the recipient is met, charity in the face of basic needs creates bonds of dependence, not those of equality. To be beholding to the good will of another for access to one of the basics of life is surely a demeaning position for a person of equal intrinsic value.

Dependence on traditional ideals fares no better. This is also likely to be an ineffective basis for meeting persons' basic needs. And even if it were effective, it would have the same demeaning feature for recipients as reliance on charity. Furthermore, although there certainly are elements in American traditions that support the establishment of a broad social guarantee of entitlement to health care, there are also strong currents in these traditions that run against it. Were this not the case, one could not account for the traditional failure of American society to institutionalize universal access to health care. One obvious American tradition that stands opposed to the right to health care is the domination of the ideology of the free market. Left to rely wholly on the weight of tradition without moral argument, claims to a right to health care might get no hearing in the current cultural and political atmosphere, where a pay-as-you-go, commodity-exchange model of health care delivery seems to dominate. Against this backdrop, placing hypothetical contractors behind a veil of ignorance is not an empty exercise, but a necessary moral distancing from the often unspoken biases within American traditions. And the conclusion that persons have fundamental rights to health care is not opposed to all American traditions. Instead, it can be thought of as an application to a technologically new and important arena of a longstanding political and moral tradition of respect for human rights.[24]

Finally, the basic view of the nonrights perspective that the recognition of a moral right to health care is somehow inimical to the values inherent in human communities must be answered. Of course, persons are shaped profoundly by the organic relationships of their communities. But communities can be authoritarian and oppressive and can therefore profoundly misshape persons. Rights are not abstractions arising outside all context, but the protections that persons need in order to guarantee that relationships in their communities contribute to the growth of rather than dwarf their individuality. Conflicts do have to be resolved by careful attention to competing interests, but among the strongest interests are persons' rights. Respecting persons and their rights requires subtlety and balance, too. No theoretical account of the basis of rights makes human judgment and practical wisdom less necessary. Love and charity are indeed important aspects of any human community. They provide a larger affective framework for justice and so give its concerns urgency and a human texture. Indeed, since the pluralistic account of the right to health care is grounded in a moral intuition that there is a duty to aid those in need, it begins with a moral fact so basic as to transcend the distinction between justice and charity. The rudimentary character of this moral knowledge that those in need must be aided is such that it is as likely a concern of charity as it is a consideration of justice. With this starting point, charity plays two roles. It is coextensive with justice, enlivening it and preventing retreat into empty abstractions. And it is larger than justice, setting goals beyond those that rights alone require. But justice must prevail in its own natural province. It sets the terms for the minimum floor of respect that persons owe one another regardless of affection and of the presence or absence of community bonds. Finally, the notion of fundamental rights of and respect for the central moral value of individuals is part of the living traditions of the United States. The implications of this part of inherited traditions must be clarified intellectually so that it can be used to correct other less morally acceptable American traditions. There is no reason why recognition of the rights of persons to needed health care cannot be an important part of the meaningfulness and sense of direction that traditions supply for a community.

Reforms

8

Market Reforms

Two different standpoints are now before us. First, from an empirical point of view, it is evident that there are significant failings in the American health care–delivery systems. Many persons, especially among black Americans, the poor, and the less educated, are underserved in light of their greater health care needs. When they are served, the quality of their care is often suspect. A shockingly high number of Americans have no health insurance or inadequate health insurance, and a large percentage of these uninsured and underinsured people are also incapable of paying for their own health care directly. And rising costs are a major concern, especially because they tend to make access problems more difficult to resolve. Second, we have examined the conceptual underpinnings of a moral right to health care and provided considerations to show why such a right should be recognized. A just society ought to provide universal access to basic health care. These two standpoints create a tension: the facts of what is the case and the ideals of what should be the case. But this sense of tension can generate the moral energy needed to reform the system in order to bring facts and ideals closer together.

Pure competition

One of the most obvious places to turn for reform of the delivery of health care in the general context of a market economy is the introduction of more market incentives into the economic exchanges of health care. Were health care delivery a more purely competitive market, so the argument might proceed, access would be expanded, prices lowered, and alternative goods and services generated. This procompetitive approach may take many forms, but generally it stresses one or both of two mechanisms. The first strategy is to make consumers of care—patients, potential patients, and purchasers of insurance—more directly involved in health care choices. This means increasing the number of consumer options and passing more of the real costs of these options along to patients and to buyers of insurance in such a way as to encourage cost-consciousness. This strategy is thus designed to enhance market performance on the demand side. The second strategy is to affect the supply side by increasing competition among providers of care. This can also take many forms, including bringing antitrust actions against such professional practices in health care as price fixing or banning advertisements, fostering the growth of for-profit health care corporations, and generally encouraging health care providers to behave more like entrepreneurs in any other business.

One set of arguments in favor of this sort of reform is simply the case for a free market in general. Free-market pricing follows from a relatively direct interplay between supply and demand. Simply put, the more that certain goods and services are wanted and the scarcer they are, the higher the price for them will rise. The less they are wanted and the more plentiful they are, the lower the price will fall. Thus market pricing creates a consumer price barrier when goods and services are rare compared with demand but, at the same time, a profit incentive for providers to enter the market. As providers enter the market, prices fall accordingly. In contrast, a consumer price incentive is created when goods and services are plentiful compared with demand but, at the same time, a profit barrier to providers, which then have an incentive to seek other types of production. As providers leave the market, prices rise. In such a competitively pure model, price will tend to arrive at a balance between the forces of consumption and of production, between the lowest price and the highest profit. This creates efficiency by curtailing the overuse of scarce items and encouraging more production of them, while stimulating the use of items in abundance and discouraging their overproduction. As a result, such a market tends to create the greatest amount of consumer satisfaction at the lowest possible production cost. If consumer satisfaction is a source of happiness, then this will generally mean the production of the greatest happiness for the greatest number at the least possible use of a society's resources. Thus this argument for market reform is both economic and moral: it is efficient and therefore serves to maximize utility.

The market approach is associated with other benefits as well. In order for producers to maximize profits, they must compete not only on price, but also on the general basis of consumer preferences. This competition tends to foster the development of quality goods and services. It also tends to promote economic creativity: generation of new goods and services, new versions of old goods and services, and new methods of marketing, selling, and advertising. All this economic creativity makes for a greater range of choice for consumers and maximizes the flexibility of providers in responding to changing market conditions. And economic creativity is closely associated with liberty. Since, in principle, this model operates only in the context of the widest possible freedom to consume, to produce, and to contract to consume and produce, the market approach promotes individual liberty. Since it is also based on personal initiative, it tends to minimize the economic role of government, again enhancing personal liberty by reducing the impact of government on individuals' choices. It is probably no coincidence that free economic markets and free political institutions developed historically at about the same time and in many of the same places.

There are also arguments for the enhanced use of the market that are specific to the present situation of health care in the United States. First, in spite of historical resistance to this point, there is nothing unethical in itself in regarding health care as a business, health care goods and services as commodities, and health care professionals as being in business for personal profit. It seems to be true that Hippocratic practitioners in ancient Greece operated for profit. Moreover, modern codes of professional ethics have acknowledged the propriety of economic self-interest on the part of physicians, so long as it does not detract from commitment to the best interests of patients.[1] In addition to fees for their services, physicians' economic self-interest may express itself in such activities as patenting surgical devices and drugs, buying ownership and stock in for-profit health care enterprises, and profiting from the prescription of drugs and the referral of patients to institutions in which the physicians have a pecuniary interest. Furthermore, even if health care is taken to be a business, pure and simple, the pursuit of profit in business is not without its own ethical constraints. Traditional moral values and obligations control the dealings of businesspeople, too. Theft, lies, and deceptive practices, for example, are as wrong in business dealings as they are in any human relationship.

In many ways, the point is moot: health care is already an industry that produces and sells commodities. Health professionals are already in business. In other words, one argument for the use of market reforms begins with an insistence on recognizing the market forces already at work in American health care delivery. Health care in the United States is no longer a cottage industry of solo-practice professionals, but is a "medical–industrial complex," dominated by large for-profit corporations, including proprietary-hospital chains, nursing homes, health maintenance organizations (HMOs), preferred-provider organizations, pharmaceutical houses, medical-supply companies, hemodialysis centers, home health care services, and free-standing emergency and surgical centers.[2] Physicians are the highest paid professional group in the country, and are more and more often salaried employees of for-profit corporations and holders of patents on medical goods and services sold for profit. Medical research and development has drawn American universities and their faculty members into partnerships with drug and biotechnology enterprises.

An interesting comment on the changing nature of the hospital economic environment is the fact that the main reference work of hospital literature, *Hospital Literature Index*, had no subject heading for "Marketing of Health Services" until 1979 and none for "Economic Competition" until 1982.[3] Each of these subject headings now has multiple entries in every volume. Increased competition in the health care marketplace has tended to blur the very distinction between not-for-profit and for-profit hospital corporations. The for-profits receive substantial public assistance through Medicare and Medicaid when they provide care to the elderly and the poor, and they generally cultivate a public-service media image. At the same time, the not-for-profits are selling tax-exempt bonds for investors' profit and are diversifying into multiple for-profit subsidiaries.[4] Among the many reasons why not-for-profit hospital corporations have come to behave more like for-profits is the marked drop in philanthropic support for these hospitals.[5] An unanticipated consequence of the establishment of Medicare and Medicaid in 1965 seems to be the widespread (and false) assumption that the government is financing the health care of all those who are unable to pay on their own and that private charity in the health care field is no longer necessary. With the needs of the poor presumably met by governmental assistance, the remainder of the health care system is thought to be able to proceed on its own, as does any other business.

Over the same period, physicians' personal charity in terms of uncompensated care or reduced fees for the poor and near poor began to fall off as their average income began to rise.[6] In 1975, the Supreme Court applied the Sherman Antitrust Act to the medical profession, charging it with restraint of trade by the prohibition of advertising in its codes of ethics.[7] Since then, health care goods and services have increasingly appeared in advertisements, just like any other commodity. Physicians are also increasingly becoming owners, stockholders, and employees in the "medical–industrial complex." During the same period, the patient-rights movement has sought and gained a more realistic contractual doctor–patient relationship, one less bound by the deference and paternalism of the recent past. In a sense, the American doctor–patient relationship has evolved over the past several generations from one bearing the marks of feudalism to one more recognizably capitalistic. And the number of malpractice lawsuits has increased dramatically as patients have sought to hold physicians more personally accountable for their failings. In short, the forces of the market are already pervasive in contemporary American health care. Market reform simply means freeing more of these forces to do the jobs they do elsewhere: increase competition and thus make goods and services available at lower prices.

The most obvious justification for more market emphasis in the health care arena is the assumption that it will lead to greater efficiency and reduced costs. The moral importance of health care cost containment is twofold. First, as we have seen, a straightforward utilitarian account is that lower costs mean greater efficiency, which, in turn, means that the most health care goods and services are made available at the least social outlay. But the second moral issue is of equal, perhaps greater, importance. No serious effort to improve access and equity in health care delivery in the United States is politically possible until the dramatic rise in health care costs is stemmed. Thus health care cost containment is a utilitarian moral achievement in itself and the prerequisite for further moral progress in expanded access and enhanced equity. But if market reform can lead to cost containment, then it has a moral justification.

Market efficiency in health care can be achieved through the same forces that promote efficiency in the sale of other commodities: price and quality competition among providers, marketing of new services, and introduction of incentives for cost-consciousness among consumers. The unbundling of health care services, price itemization, outpatient and home services where once there were only inpatient services, and the new diversity of employer insurance packages lead to greater consumer awareness of health care choices and prices. Passing on higher deductibles, co-payments, and co-insurance to consumers makes them bear more of the real cost of health care choices and thus promotes their prudent use of the system. The proliferation of prepaid health plans—such as HMOs, preferred-provider organizations, and other nontraditional practice settings—introduces both new choices for consumers and competitive price pressures on providers. The elimination of retrospective Medicare reimbursement in favor of diagnosis related groups (DRGs) and the likely adoption of this reimbursement mechanism by all third-party payers and for physicians' fees further necessitates cost-consciousness among providers. And there may never have been a more propitious time for the introduction of more market competition. The United States is in the midst of a massive increase in the number of physicians per capita; by the year 2000, the ratio will be twice what it was in 1960.[8] Market reform can help to ensure that this increase of providers works to the advantage of consumers by lowering prices and making services more widely available.[9] But the absence of market discipline combined with this dramatic increase in physicians could lead to significant inefficiencies of supply and might tend to absorb too much of the nation's resources into health care.

The use of market forces not only can work to contain prices and overutilization by promoting efficiency, but also can generate funds through the ability of the for-profit and not-for-profit health care corporations to draw on investment capital in the stock and bond markets.[10] Given the loss of major philanthropic support, the only obvious source of health care financing other than the free market is the government. But this fact introduces the final strength of market reform. Reliance on governmental funding means reliance on taxation, which, in turn, means reliance on the taking of private wealth. By contrast, raising funds in the stock and bond markets means financing health care on the basis of the free choices of investors to seek a return on their capital in both for-profit and not-for-profit health care corporations. Thus whereas governmental funding implies coercion, the market approach is based on free choice in funding. Similarly, a general reduction of the role of government in health care may be expected as a consequence of an increase in the use of the market. When the market rations access and regulates equity and quality, it does so through the operations of a multitude of individual choices without the burdens of governmental bureaucracy and interest-group politics. It also minimizes the need for government to make choices on divisive moral questions, such as abortion and the removal of technological life-support systems from those in persistent vegetative states.[11] These decisions can be left to private individuals and institutions. Generally, then, market reform in health care is consistent with greater individual liberty.

A hobbled market

But, of course, there is another side of the issue. The efficiency of the supply-and-demand model presumes an ideal situation of pure competition. Seldom is this simplifying presumption approximated in any real market. A market is often dominated by a monopoly in supply or a monopsony in demand. The real persons who constitute the forces of the pure-competition model are unequally situated at the very outset and so respond quite differently to price incentives: the poor often unable to buy, no matter how low the price; the rich often undeterred, no matter how high. The nature of a product or service sometimes is such that the consumer is unable to make competent comparisons of products or services and therefore cannot judge the relative importance of price differentials. Moreover, demand can be deliberately created or manipulated by advertisement. When this is the case, as it plainly is throughout the United States economy, no simple utilitarian evaluation of a market's moral performance is possible. A market driven by advertising is satisfying not simply preexisting demand, but also demand it has created or helped to create. It is not obvious that an economy is more efficient in a morally important sense when it cultivates demands and creates needs, even if it can then satisfy them. On the contrary, the bulk of Western philosophical wisdom seems to point in the opposite direction: that the limitation and simplification of demands and needs is the surest way to maximize happiness. And certainly, there is no utilitarian benefit, but only loss, when artificially created demands go unsatisfied, as they surely must for many who are affected by advertisements, but are unable to afford the goods and services so seductively dangled before them.

Some goods and services have important externalities, costs and benefits that do not enter into the price and profit calculations of either consumer or producer. These unrecognized costs and benefits are sometimes of significance to society as a whole, as are the public cost of air pollution and the public benefit of natural beauty in the environment. There are some goods and services whose value to the public is too important to leave to the vicissitudes of commodity exchange. National defense, basic education, religion, art, utilities, the vote, and sexual relations are or create such sensitive and basic public goods that they are either sheltered from some market forces or held outside the market economy entirely. As the earlier discussion of slavery indicates, some values are simply too great inherently to be reduced to pricing relative to other values. And liberty is a far more complex notion than simple noninterference with a wide range of consumer choices. A practical conception of liberty has to include positive freedom of access to those things that persons need to live a decent human life. Certainly, an economic system that denies or compromises positive freedom of access to life's basic necessities for those unable to pay is not beyond reproach in terms of its commitment to personal liberty, regardless of the vitality of its marketplace.

Specific difficulties with pure market reform become more evident the closer the realities of contemporary health care are examined. Surely, there are strong elements of a free market in contemporary health care in the United States, but just as clearly, the health care market is inherently defective from the perspective of the pure supply-and-demand model.[12] There have been and continue to be substantial public investments in health care, in the education of health professionals, and in health-related research. Federal and state governments have nearly monopsonistic purchasing power by virtue of paying about 40 percent of the total costs of health care in the United States.[13] Many patients are faced with provider monopoly by dint of location, method of payment, or employers' insurance decisions. Although insurance may be bought in a cool and detached moment, the need for health care itself is irregular, unpredictable, and often overriding. A patient can rarely be an effective consumer. The nearly universal payment of medical bills by third parties—private insurance companies, the government, and employer group plans—insulates the consumer from the full reality of the economic exchange in the delivery of health care. Moreover, consumers' continued purchase of first-dollar insurance coverage, through their employers or supplementally as individuals, indicates a strong preference to keep decisions about health care unaffected by immediate financial concerns.[14]

Finally, health care goods and services are nonstandard. This fact hobbles any conceivable health care marketplace in three ways. Consumers are unable to rely on others' experience as a buying guide because the factors causing disease and recovery are too complex and too unique to particular persons. Consumers are unable to test most health care products before purchase because in many cases, such as surgery, the product and the act of production are identical. Finally, consumers are unable to appraise the quality of their health care even after receiving it because the body's natural ability to heal and to limit disease processes is always an immeasurable factor in recovery or failure to recovery.

The nonstandard charcter of health care goods and services underscores the central moral role of the health care professional. Although it may not be unethical in itself for physicians, for example, to adopt the posture of the business world, there surely are negative moral consequences implied by such a choice. Since the satisfaction of the health care needs of each particular patient requires the application of a specific nonstandard treatment, patients stand in an exceptionally vulnerable position with respect to physicians. Patients rely on the vastly superior scientific knowledge, practical health care experience, and access to health care institutions that is provided by their physicians. Up to 70 percent of patients' health care expenditures—tests, drugs, surgery, referrals, and such—are under the more or less direct control of their physicians.[15] Consequently, the delivery of health care is simply not analogous to the marketing of commodities. On the contrary, effective health care delivery requires the presence of an unusually strong bond of trust between patient and physician.

Traditionally, this trust has been founded on the health care profession's commitment to the doctrine of fiduciary agency, the requirement that physicians and other health care professionals act always for the best interest of their patients and never for their own interest when it may be detrimental to a patient. Furthermore, since the possibility of generating trust in any given doctor–patient relationship relies at the start on a cultural perception of the trustworthiness of physicians in general, the profession has long required the avoidance of even the appearance of a conflict between the interests of patient and of physician.[16] No similar claim can be made for those engaged in business. In business contexts, even where traditional moral values and obligations prevail, the self-interest of the provider is

presumed to be a natural and expected part of the exchange. It is understood by both consumer and provider that the provider's self-interest sometimes does work to the direct disadvantage of the consumer; hence, the
traditional advice urging the buyer to beware. The adoption by the medical
profession of the business world view thus threatens its commitment to the
doctrine of fiduciary agency and the protection it affords to patients, who in
health care contexts find it exceptionally difficult to be truly wary of the
providers on whom they so rely.

Specifically, the increasingly commercialized practice of medicine gives
rise to overt conflicts of interest.[17] These conflicts include physicians referring their patients to for-profit hospitals or ancillary service centers of which
they are part owners,[18] physicians sharing the profit that a hospital makes
on the early discharge of their patients,[19] and physicians investing in certain
medical equipment and then prescribing its use by their patients twice as
frequently as those physicians who do not own their own equipment.[20]
Should circumstances like those come to prevail in American health care,
physicians will threaten to become "double agents," as clearly motivated for
themselves as they are for their patients.[21] Worse still, compared with the
frank self-interest of the business world, these physicians' interests are
invisible to most patients in concrete therapeutic circumstances. Patients do
not routinely have the opportunity to apply the same scrutiny and skepticism in the health care field that they do in the business environment. But as
the group behavior of physicians becomes more and more commercialized,
the more evident these conflicts of interest will become. This may help to
alert individual patients to their physicians' self-interest, but it will also
extract a large social cost. When physicians behave like businesspeople, then
even when individual physicians practice with complete integrity amid these
temptations to economic self-interest, damage will be done to public trust by
the appearance of physicians' self-interest.[22] This means that patients will
enter individual doctor–patient relationships more skeptically, be less inclined to do everything that their physicians direct, and be more willing to
sue for damages when outcomes are unfavorable.[23] Such results are not in
anyone's long-term best interest.

Furthermore, the increasingly evident business model of health care delivery will likely rob physicians of part of their own professional autonomy. In
the past, the medical profession accepted some commercial practices when
they were under physicians' control, such as ownership of proprietary
hospitals by physicians. It also accepted lay control over health care settings
in nonprofit institutions—eleemosynary hospitals with lay boards of direc-
tors, for example. But now the medical profession is faced for the first time
with the combination of both: lay control in commercialized, for-profit
settings.[24] Whether physicians can maintain their professional autonomy

over medical practice in these settings or whether they will become captives of large for-profit health care corporations is an open question at present.[25] What is already evident is that physicians are beginning to behave less like colleagues and more like competitors, a hallmark of the shift from a professional to a business ethos.[26] As this change becomes increasingly obvious, as physicians' self-interest begins to replace the more traditional altruism, the general public will probably begin to see less justification for deferring to physicians' self-regulation and will be more inclined to impose public regulation on the profession from without.[27] No one seriously expects self-interested businesspeople to be able to regulate themselves in ways that also serve the public interest.

There are also good reasons to doubt that enhanced market competition will contain health care costs. As has already been pointed out, government pays 40 percent of all health care bills. This commitment began in the mid-1960s, when almost all major hospitals were not-for-profit and the few proprietary operations were small doctors' hospitals. In the present increasingly for-profit context, this financial commitment of the government works to virtually guarantee profitability, accounting in good measure for the spread of investor-owned for-profit hospital chains, nursing homes, and hemodialysis centers, for example.[28] Having established this niche of private profit from large and predictable government entitlement programs, such as Medicare and Medicaid, these enterprises are insulated to a great extent from real market forces. Certainly, they will have to behave more competitively when greater market forces and government pressures such as DRGs come to bear, but corporations receiving such a large proportion of their income from government payments are simply not in a supply-and-demand marketplace, and they cannot be expected to behave as such. For example, it could have been expected theoretically that market discipline—price and service competition and the need to create a return on investment—would cause for-profit hospitals to be more efficient than not-for-profit hospitals. But the evidence to date is that for-profit hospitals are not more efficient; they make their profits by simply charging more than not-for-profits.[29] Obviously, if this mounting evidence is reliable, then the presence of investor-owned for-profit hospital chains increases rather than contains the overall social costs of health care. And it is revealing that the higher charges show up overwhelmingly in the ancillary, high-technology services that are used much more often in proprietary settings.[30]

These facts suggest another onerous implication of health care operated as a business. It may tend to develop and market services that offer a high return on investment, regardless of external social cost and regardless of relationship to health care needs. This portends more high-technology, acute-care–oriented health care, when the likeliest direction for cost containment is the reverse—low-technology, prevention-oriented care. And pursuit of profit in health care may even lead to outright economic waste through the production and marketing of what some commentators have called "a legion of medical hula hoops, pet rocks, and Cabbage Patch dolls."[31] Health care institutions operated for investors' profit can be expected by their very nature to follow the path of profit. This path will often lie not in the direction of satisfaction of persons' health care needs, but toward satisfaction of health-related desires, which one can expect to be more and more manipulated by advertisements. Advertising for cosmetic surgery has recently exploded across the country, for example. The continuation of this trend would take the health care–delivery system a considerable distance away from any utilitarian moral justification of market efficiency.

From the point of view of enhanced freedom, market reform may increase the freedom of some, but at the likely cost of the freedom of others. As already pointed out, the medical profession may lose some of its collective freedom as business control increases. Local communities may lose control over their own health care institutions as the pressures of profitability drive local hospitals, nursing homes, and physicians' group practices into consolidation with national chains. This may result in the replacement or diminution of the authority of local governing boards and the consequent loss of focus on local public welfare.[32] Their responsibility to stockholders will lead large for-profit corporate entities to make decisions to open or close services and whole institutions based on their own financial priorities, and not necessarily on the health care needs of the communities in which they are located. This will place additional pressure on other hospitals. "Public concern is warranted about the continued vitality and even the survival of important not-for-profit and public health care institutions—particularly those that provide large amounts of uncompensated care, and those that are valuable centers of education, research, and tertiary care."[33]

More important, freedom of access to health care goods and services will likely be compromised for those whose treatment is unprofitable. The United States remains a society of vast inequalities of wealth; the top 20 percent in income earn eleven times that of the bottom 20 percent.[34] Since health care is a superior economic good—that is, one on which more is spent as income rises—it can be expected that for-profit health care businesses will tend to cater to the more, not the less, well-to-do, since it is with them that the money and profit lie. This will mean more freedom of choice for some; health care needs, desires, and even fantasies will be well served in wealthy American suburbs, for example. But it may also mean deprivation of freedom for others; basic needs in the inner cities may continue to go unmet, for example. The poor, members of racial minorities, those with high health risks, residents of isolated areas, and those with unprofitable health care needs will likely be underserved or not served at all by a free-market system in search of profit. Evidence already suggests that for-profit hospitals, for example, provide less uncompensated care to the poor than do other hospitals and are "cream skimming" the most profitable patients.[35] Anecdotal evidence abounds of persons who cannot demonstrate ability to pay being sent away from emergency rooms at private hospitals and "dumped" on public hospitals.[36] It is only reasonable to expect that more competitive pressures in the health care marketplace will mean more of these unsavory practices. None of these concerns is based on a presumption of malice or bad faith on the part of health care entrepreneurs. The only presumption needed is that health care operated as a business will respond to the pressures that shape the world of business. There is just no economic incentive to serve certain segments of the population, in spite of their health care needs. But loss of access to health care can be a direct assault on these individuals' real exercise of freedom if it leads to needless pain, suffering, disability, and premature death. Thus market reform could lead to a worsening of conditions for those already worst off, and for those health care institutions that continue to try to serve them.

Finally, if, as has been argued, access to a decent level of basic health care is a moral right, then there is a limit in principle to the use of market reform. If the forces of the marketplace can be used to promote more efficient provision of health care, to introduce creativity, and to expand the range of real personal freedoms, then market reform can be an acceptable complement to the recognition of a moral right to health care. It can even work to enhance respect for this right, if it helps to reduce costs per unit of care, thus freeing more resources to ensure universal access and improved equity. But it can also subvert the right to health care by making access impossible for many. If health care is a right, it cannot be conditioned wholly on the ability to pay, as the pure supply-and-demand model dictates. Higher deductibles, co-payments, and co-insurance can be used legitimately to promote greater cost-consciousness among consumers and to discourage frivolous use of scarce health care resources. Cost sharing by patients might best be accomplished by basing the amount shared on a percentage of income, in order to avoid the regressive result of having the wealthy and the poor pay the same dollar amounts.[37] But these measures cannot be used to the point where they discourage satisfaction of genuine need or deny whole categories of persons access to necessary health care. The ability to pay may play a role, but a role secondary to the primary concern of seeing that the moral right to health care is respected.

Thus health care is not just another commodity; the health professions are not just businesses; and the health care system is not just a field for corporate profit in a "medical–industrial complex." Health care is primarily a person's right; health professionals are primarily fiduciary agents; and the primary goal of the health care system is to provide an important public good. This means that to one extent or another, the government must play the final role as guarantor of the right to health care.[38] Government can use the market to assist in meeting this goal, but it cannot abdicate its responsibility to the common good and to individual rights by turning over health care delivery to a for-profit mechanism bound by its nature to work against the interests of those already suffering disproportionately in American society.

In a supplementary statement to the Institute of Medicine's report *For-Profit Enterprise in Health Care*, several members of the committee that wrote the report voiced concerns similar to those expressed here. They concluded: "These concerns reinforce the implication of the committee's report that we would have little to gain, and possibly much to lose, if for-profit corporations came to dominate our health care system."[39]

9

DRGs, HMOs, and Vouchers

An alternative to straightforward market reform is market regulation or alteration in such a way as to simultaneously achieve public goals and increase marketplace efficiency. Many proposals to this effect have been made recently, and many adjustments and changes have already begun. It would be impossible to examine in detail all the many new regulatory forces in place or proposed for the delivery of health care in the United States, but a sense of the range and significance of what is possible can be gained by scrutinizing three major market alterations. Two of them—diagnosis-related group reimbursement for Medicare charges (DRGs) and prepaid group-practice plans, or health maintenance organizations (HMOs)—are already realities with growing significance. The third, the use of cash assistance programs or government vouchers for the purchase of health care for the poor, is a significant alternative proposal. Simply put, these three alternatives are an attempt to introduce governmental price controls (DRGs), a reversal of the economic incentives of medical practice (HMOs), and a facilitation of consumer sovereignty (vouchers).

Price controls

Legislation to change the method of reimbursement for Medicare charges was passed in 1983 at the congressional equivalent of the "speed of light."[1] This rapid legislative consensus was forged by dramatically rising prices in the Medicare program. Between 1967, when the program went into effect, and 1982, hospital reimbursement, which constitutes 71 percent of all Medicare costs, rose at an annual rate of about 20 percent.[2] Total Medicare expenditure in 1967 was $4.5 billion; by 1984, it totaled over $66 billion; by 1986, it reached $74.7 billion.[3] Unabated, this rate of increase threatened to bankrupt the program. It probably was the result of many factors, including an increase in the number of persons over sixty-five; a growth in enrollments from other categories of beneficiaries, including the severely disabled and those with end-stage renal disease; and an expansion of medical technology. But most of the increase is attributable to rises in the cost of a day in a hospital. This figure had gone from $670 a day in 1971 to more than $2,000 by 1984.[4]

From the DRG perspective, the primary culprit in this cost escalation is the combination of fee-for-service medicine (FFS) and the practice of Medicare's reimbursing the cost of hospital care on the basis of usual, customary, and reasonable charges. FFS medicine provides an economic incentive to do more for each patient, since it is on the basis of what is done that hospitals and physicians derive their incomes.[5] When approximately 88 percent of these charges are paid for by third parties (40 percent by the federal government), neither the hospital, the physician, nor the patient has an incentive to contain costs.[6] And when the federal government pays any Medicare bill that is deemed usual, customary, and reasonable, the consequences of the operation of these perverse economic incentives are simply passed on to the taxpayer. The reform passed in 1983 was designed to end the practice of allowing these larger and larger hospital charges to be passed on to the Medicare program by introducing price controls on federal reimbursement. These controls are of such a dramatic nature that they have led one hospital spokesman to refer to DRGs as a "punitive measure" directed at hospitals.[7]

DRG price controls are based on a packaging of all hospital charges into one figure determined by the average cost of treating patients who have the same diagnosis.[8] This amount is reimbursed to hospitals for Medicare patients with that diagnosis regardless of the actual costs involved in treating individual patients. Thus this system creates a prospective, rather than a retrospective, reimbursement scheme—one determined before, not after, treatment. If the hospital can treat the patient for less than the DRG reimbursement, it keeps the difference and thereby makes money. If it costs the hospital more to treat the patient than the DRG allows, it simply loses money. Thus this change in reimbursement creates an economic incentive for hospital efficiency, since it is clearly in the interests of hospitals to treat their Medicare patients for less money.

There are 468 DRGs. Because the full system is gradually being introduced, historical charges and regional differences still have an impact on reimbursement. But in the final system, all hospitals will be charged one national rate for each diagnosis, modified only by the hospitals' rural or urban setting (and perhaps by some continued allowance for educational costs in teaching hospitals). DRGs can also be affected by patients' length of stay, secondary diagnosis, surgery, and patients' age as it affects length of stay. An extra allowance is made for cost "outliers," those whose treatment costs exceed DRG payment by 150 percent or $12,000, whichever is greater. When this limited is reached, Medicare pays 60 percent of additional costs. But there are tight limits on the total number of outliers any hospital can claim.

The federal government is planning to extend DRG-type payment to physicians and to all providers of care to Medicare patients.[9] And other third-party payers, such as Blue Cross and Blue Shield, are beginning to adopt forms of prospective payment modeled on the DRGs. In some states, an all-payer system is already operating; that is, every third-party payer in the state reimburses prospectively.[10]

The introduction of the DRGs is a clear instance of the monopsony purchasing power of the federal government. Because the government pays 40 percent of the bills of hospital patients and public expenditures account for 53 percent of all hospital revenue, the Medicare program has been able to impose price controls on providers.[11] These controls may have contributed to a drop in hospital utilization and a shorter average length of stay, and have probably slowed the purchase of new medical technology.[12] And they have changed the economic incentives to promote efficiency in what had been an inherently inflationary system.

But there are problems with the DRG approach. First, considered only in economic terms, DRGs may not actually reduce costs in the long run. There is no evidence yet that DRGs have led to greater productivity in hospitals, only that people are using hospitals less and staying a shorter time when they do.[13] Since a DRG is paid for every hospital admission, there is a built-in incentive to admit more patients and even to discharge patients and readmit them later.[14] This may actually promote overutilization, especially in the present climate of intense competition for hospital patients. There is evidence that the DRGs have led to layoffs and changes in work assignments.[15] Of itself, this might promote efficiency; but it is also associated with increased unionization activity and a sharp rise in age- and sex-discrimination lawsuits. It is also clear that the financial pressures caused by DRGs are causing horizontal and vertical integration of health care institutions, which allows for an increase in referrals and in costs in parts of the health care system presently uncontrolled by DRGs, such as rehabilitation and psychiatric hospitals, nursing homes, and home health care agencies.[16] These institutions are increasingly operated for profit, and if the pattern established by investor-owned for-profit hospitals applies to them, profit will be made not by providing more efficient care, but by charging higher prices.[17]

Thus there is a concern that squeezing Medicare money out of hospitals will tend only to increase the costs of other kinds of care. It also seems that DRGs may tend to reduce investments by hospitals in expensive and impersonal medical technology. But they also may have a limited effect in the other direction. If a medical technology hastens the discharge of patients, for example, it may be a DRG-profitable investment. This could make patients' shortened lengths of stay even more technology intensive, thereby exacerbating one frequently criticized feature of American medicine. Finally, it is questionable in principle whether price controls can remain effective in only one sector of a massive health care economy without inflation in those prices themselves or serious economic dislocation elsewhere. The latter is predicted, for example, when DRGs become national. Since there are significant regional pricing and practicing differences, one national pricing system may mean a large interregional redistribution of resources, providing unmerited windfalls for some providers in some sections of the nation and undeserved hardships for others.[18]

Second, the system promotes prejudice against the very sick.[19] Since there is at present no DRG index for severity of illness, a hospital receives the same reimbursement for two patients with the same diagnosis, even if one is significantly more ill than the other. And cost outliers can be financially disastrous for hospitals, since the extra costs entailed by treating these persons is not reimbursed until the hospital has already absorbed a substantial loss, and the reimbursement is at a rate of only 40 percent. If FFS and usual, customary, and reasonable charges created a perverse economic incentive for hospitals, DRGs may create a perverse institutional incentive: making the very persons who most need hospital care into those patients whom hospitals will most want to avoid. This not only may create discrimination against the very sick at the point of hospital admission, but also may provide an incentive for the premature discharge of patients who may still be too sick to leave the hospital. There have been reports of elderly patients being harassed into leaving hospitals before they felt ready to go, and, obviously, if this practice occurs it can create great harm.[20] What is clear is that since the introduction of DRGs, sicker, more medically frail persons are entering nursing homes and rehabilitation centers.[21] And elderly Americans who live alone are having problems providing for their more intensive posthospital care. Even among those who have caretakers at home, new strains on families are created by having to take on unusual and demanding nursing burdens.[22]

A third difficulty with DRGs is the impact they will probably have on the medically indigent. A major means of paying for charity care and bad hospital debt has been cost shifting—that is, raising the price to paying customers to cover the costs of serving nonpaying customers.[23] Since there are up to 35 million persons in the United States with neither the private financial resources nor the health insurance to afford their own care,[24] this is a huge social problem, and cost shifting has been the widespread response. But when a large percentage of a hospital's patient charges are now controlled by DRGs and other prospective-payment methods, the use of cost shifting is limited or no longer possible. Although the burden of providing indigent care is disproportionately distributed among only about 18 percent of hospitals—predominantly public hospitals, inner-city hospitals, and teaching hospitals—the government has refused to raise DRG reimbursement for these hospitals; thus they have done very poorly under the new system.[25] Thirty percent of those cared for at large teaching hospitals, for example, have no insurance, and the DRGs have led to especially hard times for these hospitals.[26] There are reports of hospitals of all kinds charging higher admission and emergency-room fees to discourage the medically indigent, turning them away when they cannot demonstrate ability to pay, and "dumping" them on other hospitals.[27] Even those among the poor and near poor who have insurance coverage—Medicaid, for example—will be less welcome in hospitals regulated by prospective payment. Since the poor are generally less healthy, they take longer to treat. They tend to be less compliant patients, also adding to hospital length of stay. And their financial condition often makes them harder to place in other health care facilities after hospitalization. In short, the poor will generally be unprofitable patients under prospective-price-control schemes.[28] This will provide an incentive for hospitals to avoid them and to "cream skim" for the more profitable, less-sickly-in, more-quickly-out patients.[29]

Finally, there is reason to fear that the DRG system will have an untoward impact on the doctor–patient relationship. DRG pricing incentives may more and more create a conflict between physicians' loyalty to their patients and to their hospitals.[30] For example, certain diagnoses are more likely than others to be profitable for hospitals. Physicians will be pressured to use these diagnoses and, in gray areas, to "creep" always toward the most generous DRG.[31] But a questionable diagnosis not only is the first step toward possibly improper treatment, but also can harm patients by biasing their medical records in favor of more generously reimbursed and probably medically worse conditions, which, in turn, will make it more expensive for them to purchase their own insurance. Also, hospitals will be pressuring physicians to discharge their patients as soon as possible, and to discharge and readmit. There have already been frank abuses. In some hospitals, physicians' "DRG profiles" are made public to create peer pressure.[32] One hospital chain shares DRG profits with its physicians in a manner aptly described as a "kickback."[33] In the first year of the implementation of DRGs, a Senate committee documented 3,700 cases of premature discharge and generally inappropriate care due to the DRGs.[34] And there are questions about whether the professional review organizations (PROs) charged with overseeing the DRGs have their own conflict between preserving quality hospital care and cutting costs because of what appears to some as a quota system for reimbursement denials.[35]

But DRGs may well have the salutary effect of ending a system in which there simply was no incentive to be cost-conscious. The average length of a hospital stay dropped by two days between 1983 and 1984, and increases in hospital expenditures fell from 16.2 to 5.4 percent.[36] Surely something had to be done to stem the alarming increase in Medicare costs. Not only are health care resources limited in general, but those devoted by government to persons in relatively powerless social circumstances—children, the disabled, the poor, racial minorities, and rural Americans—are politically vulnerable in ways that Medicare probably is not. These constituencies would most likely have suffered first and hardest by federal health care budget tightening caused by runaway Medicare costs.

There may be other long-run benefits from prospective payments. If they are applied to physicians' fees, they may provide the government with a powerful pricing lever to increase the number of physicians in certain understaffed specialties, such as family practice and (in some areas) obstetrics and gynecology, and to attract physicians into underserved geographical areas, such as rural and inner-city practices.[37] Furthermore, the evolution of all-payer systems in several states has raised new possibilities. In these cases, industry domination of government regulation, an all-too-familiar American scenario, has been replaced by substantial public control over hospitals, with the result of significant savings.[38] In these states, the problem of financing indigent care has also been more effectively addressed by pooling hospital resources to pay for uncompensated care, by taxing insurance premiums, or by shifting costs on a systemwide scale—that is, passing the cost of indigent care through to the rates of all payers and compensating the hospitals that provide the care. From the point of view of the poor served by hospitals in these states, the all-payer prospective-reimbursement system begins to look quite a bit like an American version of national health insurance.[39]

Prepaid group practice

A second alternative approach for realizing public goals in a modified health care marketplace is to change the setting of medical practice itself. As already pointed out, part of the financial problem of contemporary health care derives from fee-for-service medicine. In this sort of practice, there is an incentive to do more because payment, whether by patient or by insurer, is based on the number and kinds of services rendered. The HMO approach reverses this economic incentive by providing a prepaid group-practice arrangement in which a periodic capitation is paid whether or not services are rendered. When services are rendered, there is no charge for covered services, and HMOs typically have comprehensive coverage. Hence the HMO acts like an insurer in which the insured is paid in kind with health care services.

One obvious benefit of this sort of practice setting is the incentive it creates to avoid overtreatment. HMOs, for example, have a hospitalization rate up to 40 percent lower than FFS practices.[40] This avoids the direct financial costs of hospitalization, but it also minimizes exposure to the 3 percent rate of noscomial infections and the average five to sixteen additional hospital days that such infections can entail.[41] Obvious, too, is the incentive of the HMO, as its name suggests, to maintain the health of its enrollees, and hence to invest in cost-effective measures of preventive health care.[42] HMOs typically have high standards of quality of care.[43] Since there is no financial barrier at the point of need for service and little or no paperwork afterward, HMOs may also enhance access. Utilization rates for the poor who join HMOs, for example, are higher than in FFS settings.[44] Finally, some are hopeful that government support for the establishment of and membership in HMOs might replace all or part of Medicare and Medicaid.[45] Were the government, for example, to pay the HMO capitations for those now entitled to either of these public programs and were there sufficient HMOs available to absorb these numbers, then the government's role in health care provision would be simplified considerably.[46] HMOs would then compete among themselves for these and other patients. Patients would have choices of various groups and coverage plans. And market efficiency would be promoted, thus lowering health care costs.

But there are difficulties with the HMO approach as well. First, although an incentive not to overtreat appears to be useful and needed in the present climate, looked at in another way, the HMO has an incentive to undertreat.[47] The HMO receives the same income whether or not it performs any services, but its expenses are determined by the nature and number of services performed. Clearly, then, the economic interest of the HMO lies in doing as little as possible. It is not obvious that, harm for harm, the harms caused by doing too much are worse than the harms caused by doing too little. This incentive to undertreat may create as great a moral conflict between the interests of physicians and of patients as does fee-for-service medicine. In one respect, the potential may be higher, since the chances for developing a personal relationship with an individual physician are lower in the HMO group practice.[48] If it is true that conflicts of interest are best avoided or dealt with in an atmosphere of mutual trust and that cultivation of this atmosphere requires a personal relationship, then the potential conflict following from the HMO incentive to undertreat may be more difficult to avoid or deal with than those conflicts typical of FFS medicine.

The manner in which undertreatment might occur is also worth examining. Although the waiting time in an HMO visit for a scheduled appointment appears to be less than the average FFS wait, scheduling the appointment itself involves longer delays in HMOs; that is, HMOs have a considerably longer lag between a patient's request for an appointment and the date of the scheduled appointment.[49] This has led some commentators to suggest that the HMO replaces the FFS financial barrier with a time barrier.[50] And since some medical conditions may be self-limiting, a delay in scheduling an appointment may mean less treatment overall. Sometimes, of course, this will be good; but sometimes not.

A larger application of this economic strategy for controlling HMO utilization is more morally worrisome. The very nature of the HMO setting determines the kinds of patients who will be served best in this arrangement. To fully exploit the benfits of a prepaid group-practice plan, patients should be well informed of the nature of the plan and of their health care needs, appreciative of the value of health care in general and preventive care in particular, sufficiently affluent to place their health care needs and desires in proper relationship to their other needs and desires, and generally assertive enough to insist on service in a system economically inclined toward less service.[51] In short, the HMO appears to be a system designed for the middle class. If, by contrast, patients are poorly informed of the plan and their health care needs, less appreciative of the value of health care and especially of prevention, driven by a host of other unfulfilled needs, and generally docile in the face of bureaucracies and systems, they could be expected to fare less well in an HMO. Unfortunately, this is a virtual description of the plight of the urban poor.[52] In fact, when California tried to use HMOs for its Medicaid population, the result was widespread fraud, abuse, and underservice for the poor.[53]

Another significant worry is that HMOs will try to enroll the young and healthy and avoid the old and sick, thus creating a patient population bound to underutilize services. But consumers who know they have ongoing health care needs, older persons and those already sick, will have an incentive to join HMOs in order to gain comprehensive coverage at a fixed rate. Thus there is a problem of adverse selection, attempted selection by the HMO of a patient population that is the opposite of those most in need and desirous of its services.[54] There are many strategies that HMOs can use to target their intended population, including offering their plans to certain employers and not to others, providing generous maternity coverage to attract young families but fewer geriatric options, and pressuring heavy users to leave the system.[55] There is some evidence that the success of HMOs to date depends to an extent on the selection of a younger, healthier, underutilizing population.[56] At the same time, there is no evidence that the preventive health care focus that might be expected from HMOs has led to any difference of morbidity rates between HMO and non-HMO populations.[57] This would also suggest that the lower hospitalization rates of HMO enrollers are not due to prevention, but to the different practice styles involved (more outpatient services, for example) and perhaps to the characteristics of the HMO population from the start.

Finally, from a straightforward economic perspective, there are some reasons to doubt the potential efficiency of the HMO alternative. First, the number of persons enrolled in HMOs, although increasing, is still too small—approximately 6 percent of the United States population—to make a large impact, even if HMOs do save money.[58] Second, there are indications that the financial savings of HMOs may be a one-time-only affair: the rate of increase in the costs of HMOs has been rising just as fast as that of FFS health care.[59] Thus whatever differential there is in costs would be realized only in the changeover from FFS- to HMO-based health care, but not in the long-term operation of HMOs. Last, historical experience with the overall performance of HMOs may not be predictive of their future performance. In the past, HMOs were run as nonprofit services by visionary individuals who were concerned to demonstrate the economic and medical benefits of health maintenance organizations in the face of close scrutiny by an overwhelmingly hostile medical profession.[60] The new HMO is more often an investor-owned for-profit enterprise in an increasingly commercialized health care environment. The generally positive track record of the HMO's economic and medical performance may, therefore, not be a useful predictor of what widespread reliance on it may entail in the future.

Certainly, if the HMO is to play a more dominant role in the future, these concerns must be addressed. Specifically, some package of minimum benefits for all HMOs will have to be insisted on in order to avoid the generation of two tiers of HMOs: an inexpensive, good-coverage plan for underutilizers; and an expensive, poor-coverage plan for those most in need of health care.[61] The general problem of adverse selection will have to be monitored. Perhaps a certain minimum mix of kinds of patients, underutilizers and overutilizers, should be established for all HMOs in order to preserve the essential social function of insurance—the sharing of risks. There will have to be a prohibition against pushing heavy users of services out of HMOs; otherwise, HMOs will fail with respect to a more obvious social function—care of the sick. Special attention will have to be paid to the alleged mismatch between the characteristics of successful HMO patients and those of the urban poor.[62] At the very least, this will require greater educational and counseling efforts within this population, so that they can be effective consumers in this system. Independent patient advocates and ombudsmen may also be required. Finally, the potential for new conflicts of interest in a less personal doctor–patient relationship must be addressed. The establishment of oversight boards composed of HMO enrollees and physicians is one possible strategy. Better yet, structuring the HMO as an enrollee- and physician-controlled nonprofit cooperative would likely be a very effective way to enhance exchanges between physicians and patients and to temper the HMO's economic incentive to undertreat. Failing these developments, the performance of for-profit HMOs should be closely scrutinized because, like investor-owned for-profit hospitals, they express the convergence of two historical ethical concerns of the medical profession: commercialization and lay control of practice.[63] In the context of a clinical environment economically pressured to avoid treatment, this combination may lead to unprecedented problems.

If these worries can be dealt with effectively, prepaid group-practice plans may have an important contribution to make in controlling the costs of health care, in curbing overutilization, and in encouraging prevention. Whether they will have a role in improving access and equity of care depends in large measure on how enrollments are financed. If, for example, enrollees must pay their own capitation, HMOs will do little to address outstanding access and equity questions in an environment of large pockets of relative poverty. But if enrollments could be subsidized so that ability to pay was not a barrier, HMOs could be part of a larger social strategy to attain justice in health care delivery. This possibility leads directly to the third approach to adjusting the health care marketplace to accommodate public goals, the use of government cash assistance programs or health care vouchers.

Cash and voucher plans

If the major barrier to access and equity in health care delivery is financial, then one obvious possible response is for the government to redistribute income from the relatively wealthy to the relatively poor. This could be done by way of a negative income tax: those above a certain income level would pay taxes according to the amount of their income, and those below that level would receive cash assistance according to their lack of income. This policy would guarantee a minimum income for all citizens, who could choose to use whatever portion of it they deemed proper to provide for their own health care—say, by buying health insurance or by enrolling in an HMO. Theoretically, the government could then get out of the welfare business, in health care and in general.[64]

Certain benefits of this approach are evident. First, it would enhance personal autonomy by providing for consumer choice.[65] If some wanted more health care, and some less, each could choose. Similarly, it would allow for wide choice among kinds of health care, fee-for-service or prepaid group practice, for example. Since it would make the consumer sovereign, persons would more likely be satisfied with this system than with any government bureaucracy. Persons know their own needs and desires best, and with cash assistance could satisfy them directly. Even if mistakes were made, such as failing to buy the insurance that turned out to be needed, consumers would still have the satisfaction of knowing that the choice, although a bad one, was at least their own. The first benefit, then, of the cash-assistance approach is that it would allow for the satisfaction of persons' basic needs without the paternalism that is implicit in social-welfare programs. Thus cash assistance combines justice with maximum individual freedom.

Second, when all the recipients of cash assistance enter the health care marketplace, a large demand would be created. This demand would call out suppliers, who would compete for this cash with alternative health care plans. Price and service competition would then tend to produce a wide array of alternative services at the lowest possible price.[66]

Third, government would be served in two ways.[67] Costs would be fixed by the setting of the initial tax rates. After the redistribution of resources, government would incur no further costs. Tax rates might be high or low, depending on a political decision about the level at which to set the minimum guaranteed income, but they would be stable and predictable. In a system of direct provision of welfare services, government costs grow according to their own logic and in ways that are hard to either predict or control. Costs increase separately for all the many parts of a welfare bureaucracy: the services themselves, other products provided, labor costs and employee benefits, equipment, construction, energy, insurance, and so on. The cash-assistance approach would pass most of this unpredictability and the problem of cost containment in general on to suppliers competing in a market. Government would also benefit by being taken out of the business of direct provision of social services. The government would be responsible solely for fair redistribution of wealth, after which the poor would take care of satisfying their own needs and desires, just as the nonpoor do. This would also relieve the government not only of welfare bureaucracies themselves, but also of all the political and moral problems they bring about. The government would no longer have to contend with various interest groups calling for more or less money in this or that welfare program; not would it be forced to confront difficult moral issues, such as whether to cover implantation of artificial hearts under Medicare or abortions under Medicaid.[68] There would be no Medicare or Medicaid, since their purposes would be served by a general income guarantee. And short of the morality dictated by law, persons would decide the right and wrong in health care issues.

But these possible benefits are more than matched by very difficult problems. First, and obviously, is the issue of how high or low to set a social minimum income supported by taxes. If it were set too low, the poor would have no other social safety net except charity, since the point of the plan is to take the government out of the welfare business. If it were set too high, resentment on the part of those whose income would be taxed and given to others would grow. But any point at which to fix a minimum income is arbitrary, for two reasons. First, there is no clean theoretical separation between needs and desires and, therefore, no objective mark at which to set income levels so as to satisfy basic needs but not extravagant desires. Second, a decent minimum not only must reflect an objective measure of what persons need, even if this could be established, but also must set it relative to the affluence of the society at hand. The more affluent the society, the higher will reasonable expectations of a minimum income rise.[69] And since a society's affluence is a varying phenomenon, the social minimum would have to be constantly reviewed and reset. Although in some sense, political and moral issues would be avoided by the cash-assistance approach, in another sense, they would be merely consolidated and thus magnified by the tax and income-assistance issue. Under this system, one can imagine considerable political and moral polarization between those who pay and those who receive.

Second, a cash-assistance program would likely create a disincentive to work among the recipients.[70] Assuming no other dramatic social changes, if income were guaranteed, cultural perspectives on the relative values of work and leisure would likely change. An experiment conducted in 1971, involving income support for over 4,500 families, showed evidence of this effect and led one analyst to conclude that a national program would result in a 29 percent reduction in the work effort of low-income workers.[71] Although it cannot be denied that much of the work available to the working poor and near poor is alienating by any humane standard, it is also plain that almost all forms of regular work serve to bring persons together in common tasks, build certain important traits of character, and provide a structure of meaningfulness for existence. And obviously, there are jobs that simply need to be done in any society. Worse still, resentment among those paying taxes would rise exponentially if a large number of recipients of income support should choose to leave the work force, and social divisions would be widened further.

There is one last, intractable difficulty with the cash-assistance approach. Under such a scheme, there would be no guarantee that recipients would use their government subsidies wisely in general or to satisfy their more basic needs in particular. Another social experiment, carried out in 1970, provides evidence of what might happen.[72] In two cities, 1,800 households were given cash assistance for three years, assistance that was intended as a supplement for the purpose of housing improvements and purchases. Although some measures were introduced to earmark the money for housing, since it was on the basis of this need that the households were selected, recipients were in essence free to spend their cash on anything they wished. In one city, only 10 percent used the money for housing; only 25 percent did so in the other. Extrapolating this result to needs in general, recipients of cash assistance might not elect to spend their money where prudence would dictate.

But what would be the appropriate public response to the imprudent recipients of income support who had exhausted all their income on non-basics and then had dire needs left unsatisfied?[73] In particular, what would be the right reaction to the persons who used none of their resources for health insurance and then showed up in need at a hospital ER? If they were treated even though unable to pay, then they would unjustly receive public assistance twice. If they were turned away, they would suffer and perhaps die in the face of the care easily capable of preventing both. Even if society were able to impose the latter option on the truly irresponsible, would the health care professionals who must actually decline readily available care be able to do so to those in genuine need? If they were capable of this, would they be the sort of committed professionals likely to be of genuine service to society as a whole? And what should be done about those whose imprudent spending followed from mental or educational incapacities? What of the children and noncompetent dependents of the competent but imprudent spendthrifts?[74] And what of the prudent but simply unlucky persons who bought reasonable insurance plans but were devastated financially by uncovered health care needs? These morally unsavory implications of the cash-assistance approach are probably sufficient to dispose of it as a serious alternative for reform of health care delivery.

A less extreme alternative in the same vein is the use of government health care vouchers. This proposal also involves taking the government out of the business of providing welfare services by redistributing income directly to the consumer. But redistribution would not be accomplished in cash, but in vouchers that could not be exchanged and could be redeemed for only the provision of health care or the purchase of health insurance. One might envision health care stamps, analogous to food stamps. This approach offers all the benefits of the cash-assistance plan, but it avoids the worst flaw of that approach, the problem of the imprudent recipient, because it targets assistance at health care. This is politically and morally important, since there is probably a clearer social consensus at present that government has a responsibility to support access to health care than that it has a duty to fix a minimum income in general. This health care targeting also could be made highly specific by eliminating voucher use for certain treatments—cosmetic rhinoplasty, for example—and by encouraging others—restricting voucher application to HMOs or insurance plans that cover a certain minimum range of services and prohibiting their use on plans that do not. This would allow the government some role in controlling the quality of health care through determination of the use of vouchers.[75] It could also in effect define a decent minimum of health care by guaranteeing access to a basic range of services covered by vouchers. This range would be reviewed and updated to include new health care services when, for example, the private purchase of insurance to cover them indicates a social consensus on their importance.[76]

But even this correction is not without difficulties. First, there remains the problem of how generous the health care voucher should be. How, for example, is the basic range of health care services to be determined?[77] Should it include organ transplantation, for example, dental care, allergy testing? Appeal to the private insurance marketplace for criteria for including and adding services might be either unhelpful or prohibitively expensive. The public insists on first-dollar insurance coverage, for example, indicating a general willingness to pay in advance to avoid having any health care decisions turn on economic factors in the context of need.[78] The larger the size of the voucher, the larger the taxation of the nonpoor, and the larger their resistance to the program. Moreover, the nonpoor would be negatively affected by vouchers beyond direct taxation. Since everyone with a voucher would enter the health care marketplace as a consumer, the effect of a generous voucher plan would be to increase demand and so bid up the price of health care services generally, for voucher and private payer alike.[79] Although vouchers might avoid the problem of the imprudent recipient because health care vouchers must be used for health care, the voucher approach would still be faced with the problem of how to deal with those whose voucher amount had been exhausted but who still needed more care. If these patients were treated anyway, vouchers would not contain costs. But could society and the health care professions tolerate the prospect of turning voucher-exhausted patients away from needed and available care?

Second, one of the central presumptions of the voucher approach is the importance of the role of the sovereign consumer, who would exercise intelligent choice and call out quality services from the market. But this model makes sense only as far as the consumer is able to make informed discriminations based on quality and price. But the failings of the health care market have already been detailed.[80] The health care consumer is too often unable to make informed judgments in this area. And other factors might limit the real range of consumers' voucher choice. One social experiment with educational vouchers reveals some of the realities that qualify the operation of the market and the reign of the consumer. A school district in California introduced a modified voucher plan from 1972 to 1977 in which public schools in the district were free to develop alternative programs to compete for student educational vouchers.[81] Although many new programs were offered, over 80 percent of parents chose to send their children to the nearest school, indicating a preference for geography or the neighborhood-school concept over markets with vouchers. Furthermore, studies of the educational effects of the experiment indicate that the use of vouchers had no overall effect on the quality of education.

If general consumer ignorance is a limitation and geographical location a factor in the potential effectiveness of health care vouchers, then there must be concern about their usefulness to the poor in America's inner cities.[82] They would most certainly have great difficulty in using this market free-dom wisely, as the abuses in the California Medicaid HMO program sug-gests. Further, the urban poor are located geographically in such a way that either the market that would serve them would be composed almost com-pletely of the urban-poor population, with the likely consequence this means for quality of care, or they would have to travel out of their commu-nities to spend their vouchers, a significant hardship for a poor and near-poor population. For the urban poor, in short, the voucher might merely "represent a ticket to purchase more second class care in degrading and dehumanizing circumstances."[83]

Finally, there are questions about the efficiency to be expected from a voucher-based market system. One commentator has estimated that drop-ping Medicare and adopting a voucher system would actually increase costs by some 10 to 20 percent because the government would have lost its monopsonistic power to control health care prices.[84] As pointed out earlier, vouchers might produce an increase in costs due to the bidding up of health care prices caused by increased demand in the market. This increased cost would then be passed on to the government in the demand for larger voucher allotments to match the higher prices. If most of the enterprises that provided the services to replace the government were run for investors' profit, as seems likely, there would be the increased cost of replacing a nonprofit public entity with profit-making private entities, with the possibil-ity, as with the investor-owned for-profit hospitals, of no corresponding increase in efficiency. And it may simply be fantasy to think that the government could retreat from the health care area without retaining a direct regulatory role, with all the political and financial costs this entails. The regulation of the use of vouchers might have to be substantial to deal with interregional pricing and practices differences, with the general prob-lem of underserved rural areas, and with the potential for fraud and patient abuse.[85] In short, the likely gains from the consolidation of government health care efforts in voucher payments for those unable to afford their own care might be offset by some other weighty costs.

In conclusion, the ideas of both cash assistance and vouchers have an attractive simplicity about them. Theoretically, they empower the poor consumer, generate efficient competition among providers, extract the government from a burdensome arena, and control health care costs. But on closer examination, this simplicity, like that of the pure market model in general, must yield to some intractable social and economic realities. Cash assistance is outright morally unacceptable because of its problem with imprudent recipients. Voucher programs have an analogous problem with the unlucky recipient. Both are overly sanguine about the possibility of attaining consumers' sovereignty in a health care market, and especially so about the urban poor. Vouchers might have some limited use where the problems outlined here can be contained, and it probably is worth experimenting to determine what those beneficial uses might be. But the moral constraints on that experimentation are strong. If persons have a moral right to some level of health care, it is a public and ultimately governmental duty to see that it is actually provided. It would be a violation of that right and that duty to remove government from this area, unless it were clearly the case that access and equity could be ensured without its active involvement. But this appears not to be the case.

10

National Health Care Plans

The final alternative to reliance on the marketplace directly or on the marketplace modified to achieve public goals is active government involvement in the financing and provision of health care. The goal is to create a national health care system that would be wholly or partly removed from market forces. The first premise of all such plans is that the health care marketplace, even when modified, fails to satisfy the important public duty of achieving some decent level of health care for all Americans as a matter of right, and that in light of this failure, there is a public, hence ultimately governmental, responsibility to create an alternative system for financing or delivering care.

Medicare and Medicaid

The major continuing commitments of this sort in the United States are, of course, Medicare and Medicaid. Medicare began in response to the failure of the market to provide affordable insurance to elderly Americans. Unlike that in comparable nations, the experience in the United States with health insurance began and has largely remained focused on employer-provided plans.[1] Commercial health insurance is thus linked in general to employment. This linkage is reinforced by tax policy, since contributions by firms are tax deductible for the employer and are not considered part of the employee's taxable income.[2] But before the introduction of Medicare, this connection between employment and health insurance meant that retired workers and their families were left unprotected unless they could afford to purchase their own health insurance. But given the health care needs of this group and their limited income, private purchase of health insurance was prohibitively expensive for most older Americans. In essence, the social function of insurance, the pooling of risks, had been defeated by a market centered on younger employed workers. This insurance market excluded from the risk pool those who were unemployed due to retirement but who were also in greater need of insurance due to age. This market failure, combined with the cultural perception that retired workers deserved better, made passage of a national program to finance the health care of Americans over age sixty-five politically feasible. The United States thus became the only nation to begin a commitment to a national health care plan with the elderly.[3] Although Medicare is not strictly an insurance scheme, inasmuch as benefits are not tied to contributions, it acts like one in the general sense that citizens pay into a pool, from which they withdraw as needed and under the conditions of the program. Many features of Medicare can be criticized, especially its limited coverage, but there is little disagreement about its success in providing enhanced security, access to care, and improved health to older Americans and to its other beneficiaries.[4]

At the same time, it was evident that the health care market was failing the poor as well. As a group, they were often unemployed or offered no health insurance benefits when employed, and, because of their poverty, they could afford neither to buy their own health insurance nor to pay for their health care directly. Thus they relied on charity or had no access to health care at all. As a result, the utilization of health care by the poor was low, and their health characteristics reflected this.[5] Medicaid was thus devised to pay for some of the health care needs of the poor. As with other welfare programs, the federal government shares the costs under Medicaid, but the individual states set eligibility criteria and administer the program. Unlike Medicare, the political feasibility of the program relied at its inception more on the absence of congressional and public attention than on a clear cultural consensus that the poor deserved better.[6] Also unlike Medicare, Medicaid is more of a mixed success. Where states have set generous eligibility standards and administered the program effectively, it has worked tolerably well. But in many states, eligibility standards fall well below federal poverty guidelines, making coverage for the poor far from adequate nationally. For example, only four out of ten women who both are of childbearing age and have an income below the United States poverty line qualify for Medicaid in their own states.[7]

Given the success but limited scope of Medicare and the limited success of Medicaid, and given the remaining gaps in the present United States health care system, especially the fact that up to 35 million Americans are uninsured,[8] three general directions for active government involvement are evident. First, the government might expand the existing Medicare and Medicaid programs. Second, some sort of universal health insurance scheme might be adopted. Third, a national health care service might be designed and implemented.

There are a great many health care needs of the elderly not covered by Medicare.[9] Excluded completely are long-term custodial nursing care, dental care, drugs purchased outside a hospital or skilled-nursing facility, eyeglasses and exams, hearing aids and exams, routine podiatry, routine physical exams, most immunizations and vaccinations, services by a detoxification facility, and any injections that can be self-administered, such as that of insulin. For covered hospitalization, Medicare charges a deductible of $520 and a co-payment of $100 per day for up to 90 days of hospitalization during a benefit period. There is a 60-day lifetime reserve of covered hospital days, but these days are nonrenewable and carry a co-payment of $260 per day. Thus in the case of a severe illness that requires 100 days of hospitalization, a Medicare beneficiary would be personally liable to the hospital for up to $4,020 ($520 deductible, $900 co-payment for the first 90 days, and $2,600 co-payment for the last 10 days). To obtain coverage for doctors' and other suppliers' bills (ambulances and medical-equipment companies, for example), beneficiaries must pay a monthly premium ($17.90 in 1987) as well as a $75 annual deductible and 20 percent co-insurance. This means, for example, that a 1987 Medicare beneficiary with $10,000 in bills from doctors and other suppliers would pay $2,290 out of pocket ($215 in premiums, $75 deductible, and $2,000 co-insurance). If this were the same individual who used 100 days in the hospital, the total annual health care bill for hospital and doctors' and other suppliers' bills not covered by Medicare would amount to $6,310 in out-of-pocket expenses. This can mean significant hardship for persons living on fixed pensions and Social Security payments. Additionally, the total costs of any eyeglasses, hearing aids, foot care, and other excluded products and services would have to be borne personally. As a result, on average, only 45 percent of the total health care bills of the elderly are paid for by Medicare.[10] Co-payments for Medicare and the prices of noncovered health care services and products are increasing at such a rate that Medicare beneficiaries now pay a greater percentage of their personal income for health care than they did before Medicare began.[11] Furthermore, in the event that an elderly person needs custodial care—that is, long-term care in a nonskilled nursing home— Medicare does not cover any of these expenses.

One solution to this problem would be to expand the coverage of Medicare and reduce the co-payments. But the costs of even maintaining the present level of coverage have inflated at such a rate that expansion of Medicare may be either prohibitively expensive, politically impossible, or both.[12] Another difficulty for this solution lies in the changing economic situation of America's elderly. Because of Social Security, private pension benefits, and personal savings, those over sixty-five are no longer among America's most poor; in fact, they may now be the least poor age group in the United States.[13] Expanding coverage to the elderly while ignoring the greater needs of others may not be the most just use of limited health care resources. Indeed, the very notion of age-based social support is morally suspicious, since even the very wealthiest of those over age sixty-five receive public assistance through Medicare. This suggests that one way of expanding Medicare coverage to the needy elderly would be to introduce means testing into the program and charge the wealthier elderly for their care at a progressive rate.

One obvious way to improve the performance of Medicaid would be to federalize the program. This would create one administration and one standard for eligibility, although both might be regionalized to account for local conditions. Eligibility, for example, might be set not by an income level for the nation, but by a national formula that would measure local costs of living in general and of health care in particular. Although cost to the program would probably rise because of the increase in the number of persons covered, the major moral benefit of federalizing Medicaid would be the enforcement of a national norm for a decent minimum level of health care that no American would have to go without. In addition, a unitary national program would save expenses as a result of the elimination of administrative duplication, could monitor fraud more effectively, and would have a monopsonistic power to control prices not unlike that which allowed Medicare to impose the DRGs.[14]

National health insurance

The second direction that more active government involvement might take would be a national health insurance program. Various plans for national health insurance have been on the American political agenda since the years of the New Deal. For many reformers, the passage of Medicare and Medicaid in 1965 was merely an incremental step in that direction.[15] By 1974, there were twenty-two proposals for national health insurance before Congress, and passage of some version seemed assured.[16] But the mid-1970s combination of inflation and recession and the rising costs of the Medicare and Medicaid programs stalled consensus on any of the proposed bills.[17]

There are several major benefits to be expected from a national insurance program. First, it would improve access to and equity of care by guaranteeing a package of minimum insurance benefits universally. Because it would ensure that care would be available when needed in the future, it also would create peace of mind in the present. And as in any insurance scheme, a national health insurance program would spread risks, sharing them at any given time between the healthy and the sick. As a national system, this last benefit would also tend to create an enhanced sense of community and underscore the social character of health and sickness. The more that risks are pooled, as in a community rating system (one premium structure for all), the more this moral benefit would be expressed, since discoverable actuarial differences among persons would be ignored for the sake of a unitary rate-and-benefit scheme.[18] This scheme tends to shift more costs to the healthy and the nonpoor and more benefits to the sick and the poor, thus helping those who are worst off. The more risks are categorized, as in experience ratings (higher premiums for those most likely to draw from the insurance pool), the less evident this benefit. Under this scheme, costs are borne in closer proportion to the use of benefits, thus shifting fewer resources toward the least well-off. If national health insurance were financed by general taxation in a progressive manner, it would also have the effect of redistribution of resources in the direction of the least well-off, since all would receive the same benefits but the wealthier would pay more for them. Whether the program were paid for by premiums or taxation, the participation of the poor could be guaranteed by the government, either through subsidies for their premiums or by virtue of the fact that the poor (should) pay little or no taxes. And an additional benefit would be the enhanced monopsony power that the government would have to control health care prices, since it would be, in effect, the single third-party payer for all health care charges.

Justification for the imposition of a mandatory insurance scheme is threefold. First, unless the scheme included at any given time a large enough number of persons paying into but not drawing from the pool, it could not be effective as a method of insurance. But if membership in the pool were not made mandatory, this could not be guaranteed. Left to voluntary participation, any national program would be defeated by adverse selection: those most likely to draw from the pool would be most likely to join it, while those most likely to pay into the pool without withdrawing would be least likely to join it. In short, the elderly, the sick, and those at high risk to be sick would join; the young and healthy would not. Premiums for a group disproportionately composed of such heavy utilizers would quickly become too high to aid the groups who now are uninsured and underinsured, thus subverting the goal of national health insurance. Commercial insurers solve this adverse-selection problem by selling policies through employer groups. When a group is composed of persons well enough to work, it is unlikely to be a group of heavy utilizers. But it is just the failure of the commercial insurance market to cover the poor not covered by Medicaid, the unemployed, and the working poor and those in smaller firms with no health care benefits offered by their employers that makes national health insurance morally attractive. Only a mandatory program of national health insurance would solve the problem of adverse selection and thus secure this moral benefit.

Second, the imposition of mandatory national health insurance can be justified by its inherent rationality. The purchase of insurance is a form of precommitment to relieve or remove the financial pressures of future decision making so as to make those choices as free from coercion and limitations as possible.[19] It is thus an investment in maintaining an enhanced range of rational choices in the future. In health care, for example, insurance allows for choices of kinds and amounts of care to be maximally free from price constraints in moments of medical need. The popularity of first-dollar coverage policies and Medigap plans to supplement Medicare show the value that many Americans attach to insulating health care decisions from financial considerations.[20] One may assume that most of those without health insurance either have failed to consider adequately the impact of the lack of insurance on future choices (recall that the age of those most likely to be uninsured is eighteen to twenty-four) or are simply unable to afford it.[21] But if this is so, neither of these causes for lack of insurance is rational. Failure to consider the future implications of choices is a hallmark of irrationality, and inability to afford to be rational is, of course, a nonrational constraint. A similar result can be reached by a different route. According to the law of marginal utility, a dollar in a context of plenty is worth less than the same dollar in the context of need. But a mandatory insurance program acts like an enforced savings plan, guaranteeing that a dollar invested outside the context of need is available when need arises. It is thus a rational plan from the utilitarian point of view of maximizing the impact of personal resources.[22] Therefore, whatever paternalism there might be in a mandatory health insurance system would be justified in the standard fashion: it would operate in the best rational interest of the insured. Insurance accomplishes this by preserving for the insured a wider range of future choices with enhanced personal resources.

Finally, a mandatory plan would create a social solution to a social problem by providing a mechanism to guarantee payment for all persons' health care needs, or at least as many of these needs as could be covered by the program. At present, our health care system is faced with the difficult human and economic issue of how to fund an unevenly distributed burden of charity care and bad debt in hospitals.[23] The practices of turning away the poor and uninsured or "dumping" them elsewhere are morally unacceptable and are dispiriting to the health care professionals forced to participate in these morally offensive activities. But the alternative of simply mandating by law that hospitals care for whoever shows up at their doors with health care needs would be unfair to those institutions struggling financially to provide the majority of this care. And it would be socially irresponsible, a bit like what it would mean to leave the total burden of national defense to those states located at the nation's borders. In such a case, a few states, by accident of their locations, would carry a social burden for all, while the rest would be "free riders." This would be just the status of hospitals providing little or no charity care, with the few doing the bulk of this good work forced by law both to provide it and to finance it for all the nation's poor. Any feasible national health insurance plan would surely have to cover the emergency and primary-care needs of all persons and so would distribute responsibility for paying for this care among all payers of premiums or taxes. Hospitals presently providing uncompensated care would then be reimbursed by the public for the public service they perform.

There are, however, objections to national health insurance. First, it obviously would entail an extension of the role and influence of government in the health care area, with a resultant increase in bureaucracy. This consequence might be minimized by government partnerships with commercial insurance carriers. But even at its minimum, there would still be more government involvement required by a national health insurance system. The only appropriate response to this objection is that this is a legitimate role of government—indeed, its responsibility. That every other industrial democracy long ago reached precisely this conclusion and has undertaken to finance its citizens' health care—without sacrifice of political liberties or a wide range of physician autonomy—is important international support for this contention.

A second problem is the so-called moral hazard of insurance—that having insurance will alter incentives in a negative direction.[24] When one is insured against the cost of health care, one may be more inclined to overuse health care services. One may eschew shopping, thus removing competitive price constraints in the market. Worst of all, one may be less inclined to care for one's own health, knowing that it can be restored at little or no cost.

These are certainly concerns that would have to be monitored and adjusted for in any mandatory national program, but they are not persuasive enough to overwhelm the goods to be had by an effective national insurance plan. Disincentives to overuse the system could be built into it; two such disincentives might be mandatory second opinions before surgery and the use of general practice "gatekeepers" to minimize unnecessary usage of hospitals and specialists. Shopping could be encouraged by providing rebates or extra coverage to those who secured less expensive services. The need for shopping might even be obviated if a DRG form of price control were a part of a national health insurance plan. Certainly, the vast monopsony power created by national health insurance would allow the government this sort of option. Finally, although other forms of insurance may well lead to less preventive care for the item insured, this is not a real threat with health insurance, since what is insured is so spontaneously valuable to the person insured. That is to say, it is unlikely that the mere fact of having health insurance would encourage irresponsibility about one's health. The realities of pain, suffering, disability, and even death are sufficient disincentives against such irresponsibility. And if these disincentives were not already effective, as in the cases of those who pursue unhealthy personal habits, the presence of health insurance would be unlikely to make a significant difference. But whatever small incentive to personal irresponsibility might follow from the moral hazard of insurance would probably be more than counterbalanced by enhanced social responsibility. If the public were paying the bill through premiums or taxation, it would likely be far more concerned about containing public-health hazards, such as ambient pollution and alcohol and tobacco abuse, and about encouraging preventive health care in general.

The real hazard of national health insurance is cost. The tremendous inflation in the Medicare and Medicaid programs in the early 1970s and the concern this engendered about the cost of a national insurance plan were probably responsible for preventing political consensus on any one plan. The inherent tendency of insurance toward cost inflation is easy to see.[25] Precisely because the choice of using health care is then insulated from financial pressures, there is a greater chance of choosing not so much a strategy to overuse when care is not needed, but a strategy to use more marginally useful, less cost-worthy treatments when care is needed. When the bill is paid for by a third party, both patient and provider have an incentive to order an additional test, for example, whose value is likely to be very small but that just might have some small diagnostic value. When this sort of incentive is multiplied throughout the tests and treatments of a nation's health care system, prices will rise and new technologies for tests and treatments will be constantly introduced with little or no assessment of their economic value. As costs rise, the pressure for enhanced insurance coverage will increase, thus confirming the cycle of health care inflation.

One response to this problem would be price controls of a DRG sort. The poor would already be protected by national health insurance, and if the incentive to avoid the very sick could be muted by the development of a severity-of-sickness index,[26] some of the most morally troubling aspects of DRGs would be removed. A second response would be to use a co-payment strategy, leaving to the patient some of the burden of paying for marginally useful tests and treatments. This would have to be done progressively to avoid the prejudice against the poor in a system of flat-fee deductibles. For example, co-payment could be based on a percentage of the patient's income. There would still remain the problem, however, of what to do about the wealthy's ability to avoid the desired impact of co-payment by buying supplemental first-dollar coverage. Perhaps such policies could be made illegal or could be highly taxed. Third, a national program of technology assessment could be devised to identify those tests and treatments that were simply not cost worthy.[27] These techniques could be excluded from coverage or only partly covered with heavy co-insurance by the patient. Finally, reimbursement policies could be framed to encourage, where appropriate, the use of general practitioners over specialists, midwives and nurses over physicians, dental assistants over dentists, outpatient clinics over hospitals, and the like. In short, cost controls could be built into the system to make national health insurance financially feasible. This must be possible, since so many other nations have done it.

In fact, in Canada, the nation that probably most resembles the United States in heritage and contemporary culture, national health insurance has helped to contain costs. From 1960 to 1965, Canada spent a larger proportion of its GNP on health care than did the United States. But after the introduction of national health insurance in Canada—phased in from 1958 to 1961, with coverage for physicians' charges beginning in 1966—this situation was reversed. The 1960 figures showed Canada spending approximately 5.5 percent of its GNP on health care, compared with about 5.3 percent for the United States. Around 1966, the Canadian percentage slipped below that of the United States. By 1980, the figures were 7.3 percent for Canada, and 9.7 percent for the United States; by the mid-1980s, approximately 8.4 percent and 10.7 percent, respectively.[28] So the proportion of its GNP that Canada spends on health care is significantly less than that of the United States, in spite of the fact that all Canadians are covered by health insurance, while 35 million Americans are not. And Canada's infant mortality and life-expectancy figures are better than those of the United States. How is this possible?

Consider the following description of the Canadian health care system.

Canada's universal health insurance system is administered by the provincial governments, gives each hospital a single annual lump sum to cover operating expenses, and pays doctors on a fee-for-service basis. Capital spending is tightly controlled, binding fee schedules are negotiated between government and physicians, and competing insurance programs are banned. A Canadian hospital has virtually no billing department and little of the internal accounting structure needed to attribute costs and charges to individual patients and physicians. Physicians' billing is simplified by the uniform insurance system. The overhead of the universal public insurance programs averages 2.5% of premium income, one-quarter of private U.S. insurers' overhead.[29]

It has been estimated that were the United States to adopt the Canadian system, overall health care costs not only would not go up, they would go down—and considerably. Administrative savings of up to $29 billion annually, or 8.2 percent of United States health spending, could be realized.[30] Since this choice would remove health care delivery from the open market, profits would be eliminated from the system, perhaps as much as $2.8 billion from health care providers and $2.1 billion from financial institutions.[31]

As one might expect, studies show that the introduction of national health insurance caused a substantial increase in access to care by Canada's least well-off groups.[32] More surprisingly, perhaps, the average income of Canadian physicians increased significantly under national health insurance, with no corresponding increase in work load.[33] This was so because national health insurance relieves Canadian doctors of the financial burdens of uncompensated care and of all the expenses associated with billing and debt collection. Finally, there is no more rationing of care in Canada than there is in the United States, the standards of care and the availability of high-technology equipment are comparable, and the Canadian public sustains its national health insurance system with enthusiastic support.[34] Plainly, then, when such a similar neighbor demonstrates what is possible, national health insurance cannot be beyond the financial reach or moral imagination of Americans.

Short of such a dramatic change in American health care, an extreme version of the co-payment strategy may be the most immediately promising direction for more active government involvement in health care delivery: universal catastrophic insurance. There is at present a widespread fear among Americans, and not an unreasonable one, of being ruined financially by a major illness. In 1977, for example, over 3 million families, or 7.6 million Americans, had out-of-pocket payments exeeding 20 percent of their family incomes.[35] Moreover, the only way that many persons in need of long-term nursing care can afford it is by "spending down"—that is, exhausting their personal resources until they are sufficiently impoverished to qualify for Medicaid.[36] Catastrophic insurance would help to address these concerns by reversing the prevailing arrangement in insurance policies, including Medicare. Present plans typically pay for the first dollar of health care expenses, minus deductibles and co-insurance, and then expire after some dollar limit is reached. A catastrophic plan would not begin until some large amount or percentage of a patient's personal income were spent on health care and then would pay the rest without dollar limitation.

One such proposal, for example, would not begin reimbursement until a patient had spent 10 percent of his or her taxable income on health care.[37] At this point, the policy would begin to pay 50 percent of the bills until 20 percent of the patient's taxable income were exhausted, after which it would pay for 100 percent of covered expenses. In essence, the requirement to spend this much of one's personal income before catastrophic insurance became effective would create the same disincentive to overuse the system as co-payments do. But unlike more conventional insurance policies, catastrophic plans would not expire when the patient needed them the most. Thus a comprehensive catastrophic plan supplementing Medicare would resolve some of the problems of the limitations in scope of the Medicare program. Furthermore, a truly comprehensive catastrophic plan might even be a morally preferable alternative to Medicare, since the question of intergenerational fairness would be addressed: everyone or every household would be assisted equally after exhausting a similar percentage of personal income on health care. This would mean replacing a dubiously justified age-based program with one based more directly on need.

Certainly, there is a possibility that catastrophic health insurance would encourage more catastrophic health care. This would be especially worrisome if it provided an incentive to use more marginally useful and expensive technologies for dying patients. In 1984, Medicare alone paid $15 billion for the care of terminally ill patients in the last six months of their lives.[38] Too much American terminal care already appears more death prolonging than life preserving. No one would want an insurance scheme that encouraged, for example, the lamentable tendency to maintain dying patients artificially in persistent vegetative states. But a national policy of catastrophic coverage might help to resolve this problem rather than worsen it if it specifically excluded coverage for medical interventions that are deemed morally extraordinary, those services that either provide no real benefit to the patient or do so only at an unacceptably high cost in suffering, inconvenience, and financial resources. In other words, the task of defining what is to be covered by national catastrophic health insurance would present an occasion for building a social consensus on appropriate levels and kinds of treatments for dying patients.

Short of implementing a program of either complete national health insurance or national catastrophic insurance, the government could do two things to help remedy the insurance gap incrementally. First, it could mandate that all employers provide to their employees an option to acquire group health insurance and establish a minimum coverage for all such employee policies. Second, it could mandate a period of time—say, one year—during which former employees would still be covered by their previous employers' group health insurance. These measures would help to address the problem of the working poor who are offered no insurance or inadequate insurance and of the unemployed, who because of our cultural choice to link health insurance with employment, now become uninsured when they become unemployed. Admittedly, these actions would place hardships on businesses, especially smaller businesses that do not offer health benefits and that compete against larger firms that already have adequate plans in place. But the response to this concern must be that it is government's duty and prerogative to establish minimum social requirements for conducting business. Just as previous generations of Americans established minimum wages and working conditions, which must have been burdensome, even impossible, for some marginally profitable businesses to satisfy, so now, a package of minimum health care benefits should be mandatory, regardless of the short-term impact on marginal businesses. The government could also take steps to insulate small businesses from the full financial impact of such new obligations by subsidizing part of the cost of their insurance plans, or by assuming all or part of the cost of continued coverage for the unemployed.

A national health care service

The third and final direction that more active government involvement might take is the establishment of a national health care service. A government health care service might take many forms, but the general idea is that government would have a direct hand in the provision and financing of health care, perhaps through a system of national hospitals and salaried health care professionals or through more direct public control over capitation, fee-for-service arrangements, and other aspects of the health care market. Such active governmental control is the norm in other industrialized democracies—from the national health services of Great Britain and Italy, to the combination of national insurance and service in Ireland, to the national health insurance and "sick funds" in France, Spain, Belgium, and Luxembourg, to the government-paid capitations in the Netherlands and Denmark, and the government-controlled "quasi-market" in West Germany.[39] In all these countries, and throughout Europe, most health care for all is either free or heavily subsidized by the government.[40] Although government intervention of this magnitude seems a politically remote possibility in the United States at present, polls indicate that the concept of a national health care service is supported by about 10 percent of the American population,[41] and legislation to set up such a system has been introduced in Congress.[42] This particular American proposal would have the federal government hire salaried health care professionals, establish national medical centers regionally, and distribute federal health care funds to publicly controlled health care agencies in local communities, districts, and regions on a per capita basis. Funding for this United States Health Service would come from a health care surtax, from the savings created by the elimination of current health care- and insurance-related tax credits for corporations and individuals, and from the funds presently spent on Medicare and Medicaid, which programs would then be unnecessary. All services would be free. Private health care outside the system would be tolerated, but not encouraged.

There are several clear benefits to be expected from a national health care service. First, and obviously, a uniform national system would be created so that, except for those who leave the system for private care when that option is available, universal access and a general equality of care would be the norm. Other national systems still have some access and equality problems stemming largely from geographical location,[43] but in general, they do a much better job of reaching all their population with a similar standard of care than is the case in the United States. One significant benefit for American health outcomes that might follow if a national health service did provide more uniform access and equity in the system could be an improvement in the average life span and in the infant mortality rate. As pointed out earlier, both of these important health indicators are worse in the United States than in most other industrial democracies that have more active government health care policies.[44] And American statistics are worse in good part because of the very bad results among America's poor and racial minorities, the infant mortality rate among black Americans being twice the rate among whites, as we have seen. These are just the least well-off groups whose health care would likely improve most under a unified national health service.[45]

Second, cost containment might be expected from a national system. Certainly, government spending on health care would increase, but the total cost of health care to the economy would likely decline. There are several reasons why this should be the case. The government would have a thorough monopsony in the health care market and could contain prices in virtually all sectors of it. Since it can be assumed that all or most of a national health service would be operated not-for-profit, the profits now taken out of the health care system would be eliminated or reduced, including those in the health insurance industry. Duplication of administration would be eliminated in favor of the efficiencies of centralization, even though significant regional and local decision making might still be desirable and achievable. The system could then be rationalized in the sense that the most cost-effective practice settings could be mandated—capitation rather than fee-for-service arrangements, for example—and the expansion of health care technology could be more rigorously controlled by system-wide cost-effectiveness assessments.[46] The massive economic and social costs of the current medical-malpractice crisis could be eliminated or reduced by government self-insurance, system-wide limitations on liability, and effective quality control on providers' performance. These controls could be imposed because, with an adequate national health care system in place, justice in health care delivery would be broadly guaranteed.

That such savings are possible is evidenced by the performance of the British National Health Service (NHS). In Great Britain, most hospitals are owned by the NHS, and physicians are paid by capitation in the case of primary-care physicians and by salary in the case of specialists. Citizens enroll with a primary-care physician, who can make referrals to specialists, who generally work in hospitals. Inflation in the British health care system has for fifteen years been one-third less than that in the United States.[47] Per capita hospital spending in Britain is half the rate in the United States.[48] Total spending on health care in Britain is almost one-third that in the United States.[49] And total health care spending as a percentage of gross domestic product is substantially less in Britain: 10.7 percent in the United States in 1984, compared with 5.9 percent in Great Britain.[50] As in the Canadian experience, much of these savings are due to differences in administration and to the nonprofit status of the NHS. One study has estimated that a changeover to a national health care service like Britain's would save Americans $65.8 billion annually: $38.4 billion on health care administration and insurance overhead, $4.9 billion on profits, $3.9 billion on marketing, and $18.6 billion in physicians' fees.[51] And this would not necessarily entail less income for physicians. As the Canadian example indicates, doctors would save on uncompensated care and on expenses related to billing, debt collection, and insurance claims. Moreover, while there surely are problems with the British NHS, such as the lengthy waiting time for elective surgery, health outcomes in terms of morbidity and mortality figures are as good as or better than those in the United States, despite less spending.

Third, as the British health statistics suggest, a national health service can deliver high-quality health care. As long as recourse to private treatment outside the system is kept to a relatively small percentage of the total health care delivered, one can expect quality service from a national system because the public demands it. Unlike welfare systems of health care, which cater to the politically powerless, a national system would serve not only the poor, but also the bulk of the middle classes, the elderly, groups organized for the care of those suffering from specific diseases, and even portions of the most wealthy. There would thus be influential and powerful forces interested in maintaining the highest possible national system of health care.

Finally, the universality of access and care provided by a national health service would enhance social solidarity and provide a focus for national sharing and mutual concern. As contemporary developed societies increase in complexity and sophistication, they come to depend less on coercion and more on cooperation.[52] Cooperation among citizens is enhanced when each feels that he or she is a valued part of a larger community, just the sort of feeling likely to be engendered by a collective commitment to a national health care service. Of all services, health care is a most appropriate one for this sort of social emphasis because of our shared biological needs and because of the ultimate existential equality of suffering and death. Although the sense of social cohesion that a national health service would likely promote is an intangible that is most properly thought of as part of a community's quality of life, it can sometimes have graphic tangible effects. The British National Health Service, for example, has been able to satisfy all its need for human blood through unpaid donors, while the United States must rely on paid "donors" and imported blood.[53] And the United States has already experienced a literal social integration from a national health care initiative: the Medicare program was instrumental in ending racial segregation in southern hospitals.[54]

There are, of course, objections to the establishment of a national health service. First, there are concerns that a national program would mean a loss by physicians of their autonomy of practice. Government control and regulations might dictate treatment options and so overrule some or many physicians' professional judgments. And this is not a concern of physicians alone. Patients, too, need independent physician advocates whose primary obligation is to them as individuals and not to any collective entity, such as the government. In short, the objection is that a national health service would interpose government into the doctor–patient relationship in a way prejudicial to the interests of physicians and patients alike.

Second, a national health service could become entangled in a skein of moral issues. Clearly, since any national plan would entail making choices about the distribution of health care resources, the government would become explicitly involved in decisions about rationing and the justice questions raised by them. One can readily envision heated political debates about the merits of public investment in one sort of technology or drug versus another, in primary versus tertiary care, in preventive versus curative medicine, on health-science research priorities, and the like. Additionally, specific moral issues in health care—such as abortion, hydration and tube feeding of the irreversibly comatose, and genetic manipulation—would become more centrally political questions, posed and resolved by government.

Finally, there is the general question of the responsiveness of a massive government bureaucracy to individual and highly specific health care needs. Would a governmental service be lethargic, paternalistic, resistant to innovation and development?[55] More to the point, perhaps, would not the nationalization of an industry, even a human service industry like health care, be incompatible with American political and economic traditions?

These are serious objections, but some of them can be answered. First, there is no evidence that physicians in nations with strong governmental health policies and democratic political institutions have lost their autonomy of practice. Evidence suggests that physicians maintain a great degree of control over other nations' health policies, over methods of practice and reimbursement, and over the character of the doctor–patient relationship.[56] In the present climate of health care commercialization and increasing number of physicians in the United States, a national health service might even offer physicians an opportunity to retain a greater measure of professional autonomy than an unregulated marketplace allows. Indeed, American physicians may soon be facing a choice of directions, a choice of historic significance: partnership with government in creating a national health care plan or absorption as employees into investor-controlled corporations. International experience provides evidence that the first road allows physicians to maintain their standing as professionals. The second road is uncharted.

Second, the moral problems alluded to earlier beset contemporary health care regardless of the mode of delivery, and the government is already actively involved in confronting them in the courts and through regulation. Addressing these problems in the context of the justice guaranteed by a national health care system might make some of them easier to resolve. Explicit rationing, for example, would be far more acceptable if all Americans were guaranteed fair equal treatment by such a system.[57] Furthermore, there is the possibility of relegating choices on some of these issues to individuals and to localities. Finally, although much of American tradition does run against public control of industry, major exceptions already include national defense, education, and many local utilities. Health care is arguably more like these other public goods than it is like a consumer commodity. And tradition, although important, is not always the best guide for solving contemporary social problems.

If the United States were disposed to experiment with a native version of a national health care service on a small scale, it might be useful to begin with a system of free care for all pregnant women and preschool children.[58] Such a "Kiddicare" program might be designed by having the government pay annual fees for each pregnant woman and every child signed up with a participating obstetrician and gynecologist, pediatrician, or family-practice physician, or with groups of such primary-care physicians. These physicians or groups would agree to provide needed comprehensive care for their enrollees for the government fee. Thus the progam would resemble a national HMO for all pregnant women and young children, with the government paying their capitations.

Costs for such an initiative would be comparatively modest. In the late

1970s, it was estimated that an annual capitation of $200 for all pregnant women and preschool children would likely attract enough providers and would cost about $7 billion per year.[59] Half this figure could be financed by removing the exemption for children on federal income tax, a reasonable trade-off. The rest would have to come from general revenues. It is important to note that of all health care, that for pregnant women and young children is among the most predictable in nature and least costly in price. Pediatric care, for example, costs one-sixth of what geriatric care costs. Additionally, the prepaid HMO-like arrangement is probably the most cost-effective practice setting. Since standards for prenatal and pediatric health care are fairly well established, the HMO incentive for undertreatment would probably not be a major problem. The free care that the system would offer, without co-payments, would help to address the health care needs of the large number of pregnant and poor teen-agers and their children. And a focus on maternal and early child care is inherently preventive in impact, thus likely to save both costs and human suffering.

This might also be a most appropriate and feasible social experiment. One of the worst statistics in American health care is the unusually high infant mortality rate among the poor and among black Americans, actually reaching Third World levels in some poverty-stricken areas of the United States.[60] These persons would likely experience the most immediate improvements in health care under Kiddicare, thus helping to save lives and improve national performance. National sympathy for children can be expected to aid the political chances of such a program. Young children, for example, can hardly be held personally accountable for their health problems. Although sympathy and release from personal responsibility are less likely for pregnant women as a group, especially unmarried pregnant women, their unborn children are both medically needy and beyond any assignment of responsibility for their circumstances. And support may come from physicians for a program of this sort, if it were combined with government protection from the soaring costs of malpractice insurance in obstetrics.

Clearly, this is only a sketch of a possible program, but it does suggest one road that a government committed to a more active role in health care delivery might take. Along with improvements in Medicare and Medicaid and schemes for national health insurance, especially universal catastrophic coverage, the creation of a United States national health service as a whole or by parts, such as Kiddicare, is an alternative for reform of the American health care system. The more active role for government that these reforms envision may seem distant from today's political agenda, but times and national priorities change. And if what we have concluded about the right to health care is accurate, then defining a more active role for government is not only a matter of political will, but also a moral obligation.

Conclusion

There are three parts to this study: an empirical investigation of the performance of the present American health care system, a conceptual exploration and defense of the concept of a moral right to health care, and an examination of alternatives for reform of the system. These parts must now be brought together.

There are, as we have seen, some significant failings in the delivery of health care in the United States. The health characteristics of black Americans and members of minority ethnic groups, of persons from low-income families, and of those with less education are decidedly worse than those of other Americans. Figures on life expectancy, infant mortality, patterns of morbidity, chronic conditions limiting daily activity, and days spent in bed due to disability indicate that to be black, poor, and less educated in America is to be subject statistically to more pain, suffering, disability, and premature death—more than other Americans, more than citizens of comparable nations, and more than is either necessary or reasonably tolerable.

Data on access to health care for these same groups show progress over the past several decades. But when these figures are corrected for the state of greater need within this population, large inequities of access are still apparent. Furthermore, we have seen evidence to support the conclusion that access to health care may not mean the same thing to all Americans. For the typical white, middle-class, well-educated American, access to care starts with a primary-care physician who is in a position to help ensure that his or her patients receive timely, appropriate, comprehensive, and continual care. In short, well-placed Americans have ready access to high-quality health care. But for disadvantaged Americans, access to health care may mean a hasty trip to the nearest hospital ER, where a similarly high quality of care cannot be guaranteed and, in light of some of the factors we have examined, seems unlikely to be secured. And there is the possibility, depending on the patient's degree of indigency and the hospital's practices, that care of any sort may be denied and the patient and problem dumped on another institution.

The programs in place to serve America's medically needy, primarily Medicare and Medicaid, have accomplished a great deal, but are still inadequate to the dimensions of the social problem. As health care costs, especially hospital costs, have escalated, Medicare has increased patient cost sharing and Medicaid has restricted enrollment. The program designed specifically for the poor, Medicaid, has been hobbled from the start by lack of popular support, widespread nonparticipation by physicians, and a state-based eligibility system that effectively excludes large portions of the poor. Many of these same individuals are not covered by health insurance. Given the central role of such coverage in guaranteeing access to needed health care, the number of Americans without any health insurance and without adequate health insurance creates the potential for a multitude of personal tragedies and the reality of a massive social problem. At the same time that Americans are apparently unwilling to underwrite adequately the health care of the poor, substantial relief for health care costs is provided to businesses and to wealthy and middle-class individuals in the potential revenue lost by employer-exclusion and employee-deduction tax policies. And, finally, there is every reason to fear that if the present national mood of commercializing health care for profit spreads and begins to dominate the delivery system, conditions for America's health care have-nots will worsen. Where is the commercial advantage in providing low-cost primary care in America's inner cities? Where is the profit in caring for those unable to pay?

The conclusion of the first part of this study, then, is that many Americans have no ready access to quality health care. Because of this, the disadvantages that already accrue to those who are black or Hispanic, poor and near poor, and less educated in the United States are multiplied by the effects of significantly worsened health characteristics. And behind this jargon of access, quality, and health characteristics is the human reality of persons' unnecessary pain, suffering, disability, and premature death.

Certainly, this situation is lamentable. But is it more than that? Is it also unjust, a violation of these persons' rights? Hence, the second focus of this work: Is there a right to health care?

Positive answers to this question have been drawn from four theories of justice and rights. Justice for rule utilitarianism is attained by any policy that maximizes the production of good consequences for those affected by the policy on average and in the long run. Persons' rights are derived from these optimum policies, so that whatever treatment is called for by a policy justified by rule utilitarianism, persons have a right to that treatment. It seems plain that were there a policy of guaranteed access to health care, much of the unnecessary pain, suffering, disability, and premature death now visited on disadvantaged Americans would be palliated and prevented. This is surely a good consequence. It might be a maximally good consequence, if the cost of a policy of guaranteed access could be contained. One method of doing so would be to guarantee access to only the health care that a reasonable and prudent person behind a veil of ignorance would choose to insure against out of his or her personal income. Such a thought experiment will not determine the details of a social guarantee of access to health care, but its implications in outline seem intuitively clear. Access to quality primary care, to basic prenatal and pediatric care, to emergency care, to some preventive and geriatric care, and to coverage against catastrophic health care bills certainly would be among the services chosen by any similarly situated person. If a policy of providing these services to all persons would achieve the best ratio of benefits to costs overall, then this is the arrangement mandated by justice. These are the kinds of health care that persons have a right to.

Egalitarian justice requires that we treat persons as equals, since from the perspective of persons' intrinsic worth, all persons are equal. The inherent dignity of each person is of incalculable value and is thus worthy of respect. Persons' rights follow directly from this dignity. Globally, persons have rights to the self-respect that is implied by the moral standing of an equal of incalculable intrinsic worth, to a range of political and interpersonal freedoms consistent with this status, and to access to the goods and services mandated by respect for the primary empirical condition of persons—their bodies and minds. It seems plain that these considerations entail a right to health care. This point is made evident by considering an egalitarian perspective on the plight of those who are so poorly served by contemporary American health care. Does one deny needed emergency treatment to a being of incalculable value? Should a being worthy of respect be dumped on the public system at risk to his or her life? Is the high death rate among American black infants tolerable when each is considered to be an intrinsically valuable being? If all are equally worthy, how can 35 million Americans be left without the insurance necessary to secure health care? These circumstances condemn themselves the moment they are juxtaposed with an egalitarian theory of equal and priceless human worth. The question left for the theory is not is there a right to health care, but to what kinds and to how much. These questions can be answered by interweaving the demands of substantive and procedural equality so that health care is distributed in general in terms of the need for it and that, if all basic needs cannot be accommodated, persons are treated equally in their chances for access to limited care.

Libertarian justice demands that persons' rational agency be protected, especially as it expresses itself in ownership. This means a special emphasis on the negative rights of noninterference that help to ensure personal liberty. The role of the government must be kept to a minimum, serving largely to prevent the use or threat of violence, fraud, and other deceptions that interfere with the free rein of rational agency and to compensate those who are victims of these harms. Within this minimal state, persons are free to appropriate nature privately and to exchange values in any fashion to which all parties to the exchange agree. Thus the preferred libertarian method of health care delivery would be a free market in which individual providers agreed with individual consumers on the terms of their provision of health care services. Outside the context of an agreement with a provider, patients and potential patients would have no positive right to health care, simply because there can be no right to what is not privately owned. But as hostile as this view is to a right to health care in general, there are three avenues left open through which a libertarian right to health care might still emerge. The entry to each is through the moral necessity to compensate those who have been treated unjustly. If persons are the victims of social factors that diminish their health, if they have been wronged in the acquisition of health care knowledge and skills, or if they have been unfairly treated in the subsequent transfers of health care expertise, they have a right to compensation. But if the actual individuals deserving of compensation are a nameless multitude of persons over generations of time, individual and specific compensatory measures are impossible. Guaranteed access to basic health care for all might then be the only reasonable way to provide a general social compensation. If this is the only practical way to correct historical injustices, then it seems to follow that even on the basis of the libertarian account, persons have a right to a guarantee of access to some level of health care.

Contractarian justice also begins with an emphasis on persons' rational agency, but with two important additions. First, persons' freedoms must be limited to be effective; but if people are to be truly free, any limitations must be self-imposed. Second, persons are inherently social, living together in communities and producing by their interactions a range of primary social goods. Hence, self-imposed limitations on freedom must be effected by all in a unanimously accepted social contract. Since such a contract is not actually feasible and since justice is an ideal in any case, the social contract is a hypothetical one, framed by equal but self-interested persons wholly unbiased by virtue of a veil of ignorance. What these hypothetical contractors would choose unanimously as the institutional arrangements for distributing the primary social goods is definitive of justice. Real persons have rights to the goods that would follow from such a just institutional arrangement. But health care would likely be among these goods if contractors agreed that it is an essential ingredient of guaranteeing equal liberty, of providing for fair equal opportunity, or of distributing wealth in order to maximize the condition of the worst-off persons in society. Depending on where contractors agreed to locate health care, the institutional arrangements for its distribution and the consequent rights to it would vary. Regardless of precisely where it were located,· it seems clear that contractors aiming to maximize their own minimum shares in life would agree to a right to health care of some sort.

When these theories of justice are viewed not as competing and mutually exclusive alternatives, but as partial insights into the nature of humans and the complex notion of justice, a pluralistic foundation for the right to health care is possible. Such an approach can be grounded on the rudimentary moral intuition that there is a general duty to aid those in need, applied to the specific context of health care. This intuition is so basic to morality as to be beyond proof, or at least to shift the burden of proof to those who deny the duty to aid. Seen thus, the theories of utilitarianism, egalitarianism, libertarianism, and contractarianism are attempts to provide a plausible interpretation of this duty in terms of persons' rights in the health care area. As long as they do not contradict one another, each can serve to reinforce the same result: that the duty to aid in health care contexts is best articulated as a moral right of access to basic health care. This result can be fleshed out by revising contractarianism to include a fourth principle—minimum security. Then a pluralistic framework for a core right to health care has four ordered parts. First is an equal liberty to be free of health interference, a right embodying both libertarian and egalitarian elements. Second is a right of access to a minimally decent standard of primary care, pegged to society's ability to afford it but provided regardless of prognosis. This right is also broadly egalitarian, but is also what contractors would agree to if it were possible that the minimum share should otherwise fall below a decent human minimum. Third is a right to curative health care, but only to the extent that normal functioning can be preserved or restored. Contractors would insist on this to guarantee fair equal opportunity, but so might a utilitarian because health care at this level would be focused where the greatest possible benefits lie. Finally, in a society recognizing these three rights, an open interpretation of the difference principle would recommend itself, leaving persons free to purchase additional health care goods, services, and amenities in a free market. This last right would be consonant with utilitarianism, since persons could seek their own happiness by choosing whether or not to invest in more health care. And because this arena would be outside any governmental commitment, it would fit with libertarian values as well.

The conclusion of the second part of this book, then, is that a moral right of access to health care ought to be recognized. But the conclusion of the first part is that many Americans have no ready access to health care. Therefore, their moral rights are being violated, and something must be done about it. That something is reform of the American health care system, which is discussed in the third part of this study. Judgments about which directions for reform are most likely to correct these injustices must be made.

It seems fairly evident that additional use of the pure market forces of supply and demand, although it might help to generate goods and services and to contain costs in some cases, is unlikely to address the social problem of limited access to health care. The creation of a purely competitive marketplace presumes too much of what clearly is not the case in the American health care system: easy entry into the market by providers, a standard good or service for sale, ability of consumers to make valid price and quality discriminations, rational control by consumers over the nature and timing of purchases, and the like. Furthermore, one might say that it is the very disposition of the American system to rely so heavily on even imperfect market mechanisms for the distribution of health care that gives rise to much of the social problem. In other words, the inability of persons to afford needed health care in the context of a pay-as-you-go commodity exchange is the primary cause of the unnecessary pain, suffering, disability, and premature death we have documented. Therefore, it is quite unlikely that more of what causes the problem can be part of the cure. Additionally, the path of market reform is also a path that threatens the ethos of the health care professions. The more that health care takes on the trappings of just another business, the more physicians, in particular, will experience overt conflicts among frank self-interest, the interests of owners of and investors in for-profit health care corporations, and their fiduciary responsibility to their patients. These conflicts may undermine public trust in American health care. But trust is an all-important and delicate dimension of the doctor–patient relationship, a dimension not best preserved in the rough-and-tumble environment of a competitive marketplace.

DRGs probably have a short-term value in containing skyrocketing hospital costs by ending the perverse economic incentives created by the combination of fee-for-service medicine and retrospective Medicare reimbursement. But they are unlikely to be a long-term solution to the wider access problem unless they are used along with other reforms, such as the all-payer prospective-payment systems that cover the hospital bills of those who cannot afford to pay them. Without such a larger framework, DRGs may serve only to harass America's elderly out of hospitals "quicker and sicker," and by doing so create other problems and expenses through the system.

HMOs probably have a brighter future, in part because they will challenge contemporary cultural patterns of overtreatment 'and in part because they lend themselves so readily to primary-care settings. The incentives to undertreat and to select young and healthy patient populations will have to be closely monitored. This is especially so when HMOs are organized for investors' profit, as they increasingly are. The real promise of HMOs, in terms of the access and equity questions we have been dealing with, probably lies in government-subsidized capitations in patient- and physician-controlled HMO cooperatives. Then the poor would be ensured an entry into the primary-care system, and the untoward economic incentives of HMOs would be muted by a patient-oriented nonprofit operation.

The use of cash income supplements in place of any public welfare effort is doomed from the start by the intractable moral dilemma of the imprudent recipient. There simply is no happy resolution to the problem of responding to the health care needs of those whose cash assistance has been wasted or otherwise exhausted. The alternative of providing vouchers designed specifically for exchange for health care narrows this difficulty a bit, but we are still faced with essentially the same dilemma by persons whose health care needs outstrip the size of their vouchers. Society must then either provide assistance twice or refuse the needed care; neither choice is a good one. For this reason, vouchers will probably not play a major role in addressing the social problems at hand.

The likeliest route for successful reform of the system in light of persons' right to health care is for more active government intervention in health care delivery. Major moral accomplishments followed previous government interventions, Medicare and Medicaid in particular, and this is the direction every other industrial democracy in the world has taken. Moreover, to call for more government action is simply to state that a collective responsibility ought to be discharged collectively. Immediate short-range government actions could make significant differences. If means testing were introduced into Medicare so that the most wealthy among the elderly paid most or more of their own health care costs, the program might be arranged to be more generous to those among its beneficiaries who need support the most. And it would help to mitigate the morally suspicious use of age as a category of entitlement. Medicaid should be federalized and a national minimum health care floor created such that no American is allowed to fall below it. Support for custodial care of the elderly and infirm should be provided for separately, perhaps through Medicare, perhaps by other insurance mechanisms. But it should not be permitted to bleed the Medicaid program, whose natural beneficiaries should be America's lifelong poor. And government should mandate a package of minimum health care benefits for all employees and continued coverage for some period for those who become unemployed.

National health insurance is too obvious and too important an idea to deserve the neglect it now receives. Were every American covered to some extent by health insurance, most of the problems detailed in this book would not exist, nor would the pain, suffering, disability, and premature death they represent. The cost to the government of such a program would, of course, be a major problem, but in principle there is no reason why benefits could not be arranged to encourage savings. The Canadian example suggests that overall health care costs might well decrease under a national health insurance plan. And the truly expensive health care services could simply be left uncovered by the national policy. It is not clear morally that society is obliged to underwrite heart transplants, for example, but no morally decent advanced society can fail to ensure that all its infants have access to routine pediatric care. That many Americans do not have access to such rudimentary health care because of lack of insurance is the major moral argument for national health insurance. A step in this direction, and one that would resolve a great deal of anxiety, is a national program of catastrophic insurance. With appropriate disincentives against the use of services that are not cost worthy, national catastrophic-insurance coverage could be an affordable social response to the devastating financial consequences that illness and injury can often bring.

A United States health care service seems so politically improbable at present as to make even discussion of it appear otiose. But if access to a decent level of health care is a right, provision of that care is a public duty. Furthermore, if the care of the health of a nation's citizens is or creates a public good, then the implementation of a public network of health care delivery designed to solve the social problems of access and equity is not an unreasonable direction to take. The point is clearer, perhaps, when reversed in an analogous area. Given the public good of national defense, would it make sense to leave the functions of the armed forces to the marketplace, even to a regulated marketplace? Then, if protection against foreign enemies so obviously requires a national system of defense, should not defense against the realities of unnecessary pain, suffering, disability, and premature death faced by millions of Americans require a similar national system? And to extend the analogy, just as there is little concern in general about the overall quality of the American military system, so there is no reason in principle to deny that a United States health service could deliver high-quality health care. Certainly, the overwhelming popularity of the British National Health Service with the people it serves is an empirical argument in support of this contention. Moreover, the changing character of marketplace incentives and the dramatic increase in the number of American physicians may well converge to alter the medical profession's longtime resistance to a national system of health care delivery.

It may be useful in closing to relate these questions of health care policies more closely to the four-part right to health care argued for earlier. Although considerable modesty is called for when moving from theory to practical policy proposals, laying out these rights and reforms together may serve to sharpen understanding of each. The first right is the negative right of health noninterference. Little from the discussion of policy reform is applicable to this right, except to observe that it requires government commitment to compensation for wrongfully diminished health status.

The second right is to access to basic primary health care, including prenatal and pediatric care, and some geriatric and preventive care. Here national health insurance might be an effective strategy, insuring for only highly personal, low-technology health care, regardless of prognosis. Or the government could arrange to subsidize in a progressive manner the capitations for membership in primary-care–oriented HMOs for all Americans. This would also be the level of health care right for which a national health care service might be a practical solution, a national HMO with all capitation paid for through progressive taxation. A useful experiment would be a national health care service based on the "Kiddicare" concept, one designed to provide free primary care for all pregnant women and preschool children. This would be a small start, with manageable financing and with a population representing an exceptionally strong moral demand.

The third right is to more extensive curative health care, to the extent that it is likely to preserve or restore functioning typical for a normal member of the species. Here we are considering high-technology, very expensive care. A combination of DRGs to control hospital costs and catastrophic health insurance to guarantee that inability to pay is not an insuperable barrier might help ensure this right. Persons might then make their curative health care choices for themselves, and exhaust a similar percentage of their personal resources before public insurance provided assistance. And very expensive as well as marginally useful services could be excluded and left to individuals' own resources entirely.

Finally, the last right is to dispose of additional justly acquired income on other health care goods and services and on amenities. Although it is unlikely that a distribution of wealth justified by the difference principle could be approximated in American society in the foreseeable future, were the first three elements of the right to health care recognized morally and enforced legally, American society would be broadly just from the point of view of health care distribution. Given that, the freedom to dispose of other income in a health care marketplace would be an individual's libertarian right. This would also create a field for social experimentation on alternative methods of health care and health care delivery, which just might have some long-term utility.

These, of course, are tentative policy suggestions. Every one of these options involves a great wealth of empirical detail, only the broadest outline of which has been described here. But what is not tentative is this: there are many, many Americans, especially among those already seriously disadvantaged in other ways, who are effectively denied the full benefits of modern health care. They have a moral right of access to a decent level of that care, and that they are now without it is a violation of their rights and an indictment of American society. They represent a large and unconscionable pocket of health care poverty in the midst of America's health care affluence. Reform of the health care system is therefore a moral necessity. Accomplishing this task will require careful attention to the realities of the present system, to the rights of all persons, and to the alternative directions that reform might take.

Notes

1. Some American Health Care Realities

1. David Crozier, "Health Status and Medical Care Utilization," *Health Affairs* 3 (Spring 1984): 116.
2. "Key U.S. Health Indicators Show Some Continued Improvement," *The Nation's Health* (March 1986): 4.
3. Ibid., p. 1; "Health Care for the Poor in 1985," *Clearinghouse Review* 19, no. 9 (January 1986): 957.
4. Crozier, "Health Status," p. 116.
5. Robert Pear, "Minorities Seen as Still Lagging in Health Status," *New York Times*, 17 October 1985, p. A16. The DHHS report states that black, Hispanic, and native Americans "have not benefited fully or equitably from the fruits" of modern health care.
6. Centers for Disease Control, "Annual Summary 1983: Reported Morbidity and Mortality in the United States," *Morbidity and Mortality Weekly Report* 32, no. 54 (December 1984): 64, 99.
7. President's Commission for the Study of Ethical Problems in Medicine and Biomedical and Behavioral Research, *Securing Access to Health Care* (Washington, D.C.: Government Printing Office, 1983), 1: 70.
8. All these figures are in Peter Ries, U.S. Department of Health and Human Services, *Health Characteristics According to Family and Personal Income*, Vital and Health Statistics, series 10, no. 14 (January 1985): 9–21. On the reliability of self-assessed health status, see p. 10.
9. All these figures are in ibid., p. 6.
10. Marjorie J. Robertson and Michael R. Cousineau, "Health Status and Access to Health Services Among the Urban Homeless," *American Journal of Public Health* 76, no. 5 (May 1986): 561–562.
11. All these figures are in Department of Health and Human Services, *Health Characteristics*, pp. 6–21.
12. Ibid., pp. 25–37.
13. Walter J. McNerney, "Two-Tier System of Health Care," *The Hospital Research and Educational Trust* (1983): 3.
14. The data in this paragraph are based on Crozier, "Health Status," pp. 114–118.
15. President's Commission, *Securing Access*, 1: 54.
16. Nicole Lurie et al., "Termination of Medi-Cal Benefits," *New England Journal of Medicine*, 8 May (1986) 1266–1268.

17. *Updated Report on Access to Health Care for the American People*, The Robert Wood Johnson Foundation Special Report, no. 1 (1983), p. 5.
18. Department of Health and Human Services, *Health Characteristics*, p. 15.
19. *Updated Report*, p. 5.
20. Department of Health and Human Services, *Health Characteristics*, p. 15.
21. Ibid.
22. Sr. Amata Miller, "The Economic Realities of Universal Access to Health Care," in *Justice and Health Care*, ed. Margaret Kelly (St. Louis: Catholic Health Association, 1985), p. 113.
23. Paul Starr, "Medical Care and the Pursuit of Equality in America," in *Securing Access to Health Care*, ed. President's Commission for the Study of Ethical Problems in Medicine and Biomedical and Behavioral Research (Washington, D.C.: Government Printing Office, 1983), 2: 20.
24. Ibid., 2: 21.
25. President's Commission, *Securing Access*, 1: 68.
26. Ibid., 1: 84.
27. Ibid., 1: 81.
28. Ibid., 1: 82.
29. All these figures are in *Updated Report*, p. 6.
30. For an analysis of health care for the inner-city poor in five American cities, see Edith M. Davis and Michael L. Millman, eds., *Health Care for the Urban Poor* (Totowa, N.J.: Rowman and Allanheld, 1983).
31. Gerald R. Connor, "The Medicaid Program in Transition," in *Securing Access to Health Care*, ed. President's Commission for the Study of Ethical Problems in Medicine and Biomedical and Behavioral Research (Washington, D.C.: Government Printing Office, 1983), 3: 90–93.
32. Karen Davis and Diane Rowland, "Uninsured and Underserved: Inequities in Health Care in the U.S.," in *Securing Access to Health Care*, ed. President's Commission for the Study of Ethical Problems in Medicine and Biomedical and Behavioral Research (Washington, D.C.: Government Printing Office, 1983), 3: 61.
33. "Health Care for the Poor," p. 955.
34. John Iglehart, "Early Experience with Prospective Payment of Hospitals," *New England Journal of Medicine* 29 May 1986, p. 1460.
35. President's Commission, *Securing Access*, 1: 156–158. The potential for conflict between the interests of the poor and of the elderly is addressed in Michael Whitcomb, "Health Care for the Poor," *New England Journal of Medicine*, 6 November 1986, pp. 1220–1222.
36. Charles J. Fahey, "The Infirm Elderly: Their Care and an Agenda for All Segments of Society," *Vital Issues* 31, no. 10 (June 1982): 4–5.
37. President's Commission, *Securing Access*, 1: 87.
38. Leon Wyszewianski and Avedis Donabedian, "Equity in the Distribution of Quality of Care," in *Securing Access to Health Care*, ed. President's Commission for the Study of Ethical Problems in Medicine and Biomedical and Behavioral Research (Washington, D.C.: Government Printing Office, 1983), 3: 149.
39. Karen Davis et al., "Is Cost Containment Working?" *Health Affairs* 4 (Fall 1985): 90; Donald Cohodes, "America: The Home of the Free, the Land of the Uninsured," *Inquiry*, 23 (Fall 1986): 227.
40. All these figures are in *Updated Report*, p. 7.
41. Davis and Rowland, "Uninsured and Underserved," p. 59. Lack of health insurance is also a problem for the more than 700,000 Native Americans in urban areas outside reservations (Jerilyn DeCoteau, "Access of Urban Indians to Health Care," *Clearinghouse Review* 20, no. 4 (Summer 1986]: 402–409).
42. All these figures are in Department of Health and Human Services, *Health Characteristics*, pp. 24–37.
43. The point that having health insurance is largely a matter of luck is made by Davis and

Rowland, "Uninsured and Underserved," p. 62, and is endorsed by the President's Commission, *Securing Access*, 1: 100.

44. President's Commission, *Securing Access*, 1: 101.

45. U.S. Congress, House Committee on Energy and Commerce, *Hearings on Medicaid Cutbacks on Infant Care*, 97th Cong., 1st session, 27 July 1981.

46. Robert L. Schiff et al., "Transfers to a Public Hospital," *New England Journal of Medicine*, 27 February 1986, p. 552.

47. Judith Feder, Jack Hadley, and Ross Mullner, "Falling Through the Cracks: Poverty, Insurance Coverage, and Hospital Care for the Poor, 1980 and 1982," *Milbank Memorial Fund Quarterly* 62, no. 4, (Fall 1984): 545.

48. The AHA also estimates that physicians in the United States provided $2.9 billion worth of uncompensated care in 1982 (Cohodes, "America," pp. 228–229).

49. Jane Perkins, "The Effects of Health Care Cost Containment on the Poor: An Overview," *Clearinghouse Review* 19, no. 8 (December 1985): 833. Congress insisted on the enhanced allowance and mandated it by law in 1985 (Iglehart, "Early Experience," p. 1463).

50. Feder, Hadley, and Mullner, "Falling Through the Cracks," p. 545.

51. Miller, "Economic Realities," p. 123.

52. All these figures are in President's Commission, *Securing Access*, 1: 74–76.

53. Ibid., 1: 70–71.

54. For an overview of some of these issues, see Nancy E. Waxler, "The Culture of Medicine Among American Minority Groups," in *Justice and Health Care*, ed. Margaret Kelly (St. Louis: Catholic Health Association, 1985), pp. 91–108.

55. President's Commission, *Securing Access*, 1: 58–59.

56. John L. S. Holloman, Jr., "Access to Health Care," in *Securing Access to Health Care*, ed. President's Commission for the Study of Ethical Problems in Medicine and Biomedical and Behavioral Research (Washington, D.C.: Government Printing Office, 1983), 2: 86.

57. Ibid., 2: 94.

58. Ibid., 2: 87.

59. Wyszewianski and Donabedian, "Equity in the Distribution of Quality of Care," p. 160.

60. Holloman, "Access to Health Care," p. 87.

61. Henry J. Aaron and William B. Schwartz, *The Painful Prescription: Rationing Hospital Care* (Washington, D.C.: Brookings Institution, 1984), p. 3.

62. James A. Reuter, "Health Care Expenditures and Prices," in *Issue Brief* of Congressional Research Service, The Library of Congress, 9 September 1985, pp. 2–4.

63. Janet Pernice Lundy, "Health Care Cost Containment," in *Issue Brief* of Congressional Research Service, The Library of Congress, 23 October 1985, p. 1.

64. Ibid., pp. 1–4.

65. Miller, "Economic Realities," p. 110. It is also interesting to note that from 1981 to 1986, defense spending in the United States increased from 22 to 26.3 percent of federal expenditures, while the percentage spent on Medicare dropped from 7.6 to 7.1 (Iglehart, "Early Experience," p. 1460).

66. Congressional Budget Office, *Reducing the Deficit: Spending and Revenue Options*, 1985 Annual Report, February 1985. In fiscal 1986, Medicare covered health care costs for 29 million elderly and 3 million disabled people at costs of $48.5 billion to hospitals, $24.5 billion to physicians, and $1.7 billion for administration (Iglehart, "Early Experience," p. 1461).

67. Davis et al., "Is Cost Containment Working?" pp. 82–92.

68. Davis and Rowland, "Uninsured and Underserved," p. 74.

69. Kenneth Bacon, "A Move Toward Lower Taxes for the Poor," *Wall Street Journal*, 30 December 1985, p. 1.

70. President's Commission, *Securing Access*, 1: 160–169.

71. The President's Commission found this pattern of expenditures "difficult to justify from an ethical standpoint" (Ibid., 1: 167).

72. Perkins, "Effects of Health Care Cost Containment," p. 843.

73. All these figures are in Jane Stein, "Industry's New Bottom Line on Health Care Costs: Is Less Better?" *Hastings Center Report* 15, no. 5 (October 1985): 14–18.
74. Gerald Anderson, "National Medical Care Spending," *Health Affairs* 5 (Fall 1986): 130.
75. Eli Ginzberg, "The Restructuring of U.S. Health Care," *Inquiry* 22 (Fall 1985): 277.
76. J. Warren Salmon, "Profit and Health Care: Trends in Corporatization and Proprietization," *International Journal of Health Services* 15, no. 3 (1985): 396, 405–410.
77. Perkins, "Effects of Health Care Cost Containment," p. 844.
78. Ginzberg, "Restructuring," p. 275.
79. Paul T. Menzel, *Medical Costs, Moral Choices* (New Haven, Conn.: Yale University Press, 1983), pp. 213–214.
80. Reuter, "Health Care Expenditures and Prices," p. 2.

2. A Right to Health Care

1. Tom L. Beauchamp and Ruth R. Faden, "The Right to Health and the Right to Health Care," *Journal of Medicine and Philosophy* 4, no. 2 (June 1979): 119.
2. Nora K. Bell, "The Scarcity of Medical Resources: Are There Rights to Health Care?" *Journal of Medicine and Philosophy* 4, no. 2 (June 1979): 166.
3. Henry Shue, *Basic Rights* (Princeton, N.J.: Princeton University Press, 1980), p. 13.
4. Joel Feinberg, "The Nature and Value of Rights," in *Rights, Justice, and the Bounds of Liberty* (Princeton, N.J.: Princeton University Press, 1980), p. 143. The exceptions to the correlativity thesis are "duties" of charity and those imposed by morally gratuitous personal commitments.
5. See, for example, Beauchamp and Faden, "Right to Health," p. 120.
6. Feinberg, "Nature and Value of Rights," p. 151.
7. President's Commission for the Study of Ethical Problems in Medicine and Biomedical and Behavioral Research, *Securing Access to Health Care* (Washington, D.C.: Government Printing Office, 1983), 1: 33.
8. Thomas H. Murray, "The Final, Anticlamactic Rule on Baby Doe," *Hastings Center Report* 15, no. 3 (June 1985): pp. 5–9.
9. Charles J. Dougherty, "The Right to Health Care: First Aid in the Emergency Room," *Public Law Forum* 4, no. 1 (1984): 101–128.
10. Article 25(1) of the Universal Declaration of Human Rights, adopted by the United Nations in 1948, states: "Everyone has the right to a standard of living adequate for the well-being of himself and his family, including food, clothing, housing, and medical care and necessary social services and the right to security in the event of unemployment, sickness, disability, widowhood, old age, or other lack of livelihood in circumstances beyond his control" (Ian Browlie, ed., *Basic Documents on Human Rights* [Oxford: Oxford University Press, 1981], p. 26).
11. John L. S. Holloman, Jr., *Securing Access to Health Care* in President's Commission for the Study of Ethical Problems in Medicine and Biomedical and Behavioral Research (Washington, D.C.: Government Printing Office, 1983), 2: p. 83.
12. Beauchamp and Faden, "Right to Health," p. 127; Peter Singer, "Freedoms and Utilities in the Distribution of Health Care," in *Ethics and Health Policy*, ed. Robert M. Veatch and Roy Branson (Cambridge, Mass.: Ballinger, 1976), pp. 175–193.
13. Sr. Amata Miller, "The Economic Realities of Universal Access to Health Care," in *Justice and Health Care*, ed. Margaret Kelly (St. Louis: Catholic Health Association, 1985), p. 123.
14. The plan for the British National Health Service was used in war propaganda in 1942 to boost morale and demonstrate the superiority of the British way of life. Its establishment in 1948 can be seen as Britain's reward to itself after the collective sacrifices made during World War II. (Henry J. Aaron and William B. Schwartz, *The Painful Prescription: Rationing Hospital Care* [Washington, D.C.: Brookings Institution, 1984], p. 13).
15. Robert M. Veatch, *A Theory of Medical Ethics* (New York: Basic Books, 1981), pp. 264–276.

16. John Arras and Andrew Jameton, "Medical Individualism and the Right to Health Care," in *Intervention and Reflection*, 2d ed., ed. Ronald Munson (Belmont, Calif.: Wadsworth, 1983), pp. 541–552.

17. Frederick S. Carney, "Justice and Health Care: A Theological Review," in *Justice and Health Care*, ed. Earl Shelp (Dordrecht, Netherlands: Reidel, 1981), pp. 37–50.

18. This approach is indebted generally to John Rawls, *A Theory of Justice* (Cambridge, Mass.: Harvard University Press, 1971), but is more directly based on Ronald Green, "Health Care and Justice in Contract Theory Perspective," in *Ethics and Health Policy*, ed. Robert M. Veatch and Roy Branson (Cambridge, Mass.: Ballinger, 1976), pp. 111–126, and Norman Daniels, *Just Health Care* (Cambridge: Cambridge University Press, 1985).

19. Robert Nozick, *Anarchy, State, and Utopia* (New York: Basic Books, 1974).

20. Robert M. Sade, "Medical Care as a Right: A Refutation," *New England Journal of Medicine*, 2 December 1971, pp. 1288–1292.

21. Allen Buchanan, "The Right to a Decent Minimum of Health Care," *Philosophy and Public Affairs* 13, no. 1 (Winter 1984): 69.

3. Utilitarianism

1. For other perspectives on utilitarianism, see John Stuart Mill, *Utilitarianism*, ed. Samuel Gorovitz (Indianapolis: Bobbs-Merrill, 1971); David Lyons, *Forms and Limits of Utilitarianism* (Oxford: Clarendon Press, 1965); J. J. C. Smart and Bernard Williams, eds., *Utilitarianism, For and Against* (Cambridge: Cambridge University Press, 1973); and Amartya Sen, ed., *Utilitarianism and Beyond* (Cambridge: Cambridge University Press, 1982).

2. Tom L. Beauchamp and James F. Childress, *Principles of Biomedical Ethics* (New York: Oxford University Press, 1979), pp. 188–198.

3. "These facts [pain, disability, death] are utterly sufficient to explain the specialness of health and health care" (Lawrence Stern, "Opportunity and Health Care: Criticisms and Suggestions," *Journal of Medicine and Philosophy* 8 [1983]: 346).

4. Laurence B. McCullough, "Justice and Health Care: Historical Perspectives and Precedents," in *Justice and Health Care*, ed. Earl Shelp (Dordrecht, Netherlands: Reidel, 1981), pp. 51–71.

5. See, for example, Carl Wellman, *Welfare Rights* (Totowa, N.J.: Rowman and Littlefield, 1982), pp. 64–76.

6. Daniel Wikler, "Philosophical Perspectives on Access to Health Care: An Introduction," in *Securing Access to Health Care*, ed. President's Commission for the Study of Ethical Problems in Medicine and Biomedical and Behavioral Research (Washington, D.C.: Government Printing Office, 1983), 2: 124–129.

7. "A state which dwarfs its men, in order that they may be more docile instruments in its hands even for beneficial purposes—will find that with small men no great thing can really be accomplished" (John Stuart Mill, *On Liberty*, ed. Elizabeth Rappaport [Indianapolis: Hackett, 1978], p. 113). See also Victor Fuchs, "Economics, Health, and Post-Industrial Society," *Milbank Memorial Fund Quarterly* 57, no. 2 (Spring 1979): 165–181.

8. Peter Singer, "Freedoms and Utilities in the Distribution of Health Care," in *Ethics and Health Policy*, ed. Robert M. Veatch and Roy Branson (Cambridge, Mass.: Ballinger, 1976), pp. 188–193.

9. Henry J. Aaron and William B. Schwartz, *The Painful Prescription: Rationing Hospital Care* (Washington, D.C.: Brookings Institution, 1984), p. 14.

10. Allan Gibbard, "The Prospective Pareto Principle and Equity of Access to Health Care," in *Securing Access to Health Care*, ed. President's Commission for the Study of Ethical Problems in Medicine and Biomedical and Behavioral Research (Washington, D.C.: Government Printing Office, 1983), 2: 173–174.

11. Jerry Avorn, "Needs, Wants, Demands, and Interests," in *In Search of Equity*, ed. Ronald Bayer, Arthur Caplan, and Norman Daniels (New York: Plenum Press, 1983), pp. 183–197.

12. For a discussion of the price of human life, see Paul T. Menzel, *Medical Costs, Moral Choices* (New Haven, Conn.: Yale University Press, 1983), pp. 24–55.
13. Gibbard, "Prospective Pareto Principle." For an opposing view, see Allen Buchanan, "The Right to a Decent Minimum of Health Care," *Philosophy and Public Affairs* 13, no. 1 (Winter 1984): 55–78.
14. Charles Fried, "Equality and Rights in Medical Care," *Hastings Center Report* 6 (February 1976): 29–34.
15. A Massachusetts task force estimated the total cost of one liver transplant at $238,000 in 1983 (Howard S. Schwartz, "Bioethical and Legal Considerations in Increasing the Supply of Transplantable Organs: From UAGA to 'Baby Fae,'" *American Journal of Law and Medicine* 10, no. 4 [Winter 1985]: 403).
16. The following scheme is indebted to Gibbard, "Prospective Pareto Principle."
17. Ibid., p. 174.
18. Edmund D. Pellegrino and David C. Thomasma, *Philosophical Basis of Medical Practice* (New York: Oxford University Press, 1981), pp. 223–243.
19. Albert Weale, "Statistical Lives and the Principle of Maximum Benefit," *Journal of Medical Ethics* 5, no. 4 (December 1979): 185–195.

4. Egalitarianism

1. This discussion is indebted to Immanuel Kant, especially *Grounding for the Metaphysics of Morals*, trans. James W. Ellington (Indianapolis: Hackett, 1981).
2. David C. Thomasma, "An Apology for the Value of Human Lives," *Hospital Progress* 63, no. 3 (April 1982): 49–52, 68.
3. Although he was a vehement opponent of egalitarianism, Friedrich Nietzsche made this point succinctly: "Esteeming itself is of all esteemed things the most estimable treasure. Through esteeming alone is there value: and without esteeming, the nut of existence would be hollow" (*Thus Spoke Zarathustra*, in *The Portable Nietzsche*, ed. Walter Kaufmann [New York: Penguin Books, 1983], p. 171).
4. Charles J. Dougherty, *Ideal, Fact, and Medicine* (Lanham, Md.: University Press of America, 1985), especially chap. 3.
5. Charles Fried, "Equality and Rights in Medical Care," *Hastings Center Report* 6 (February 1976): 29–34, and *Right and Wrong* (Cambridge, Mass.: Harvard University Press, 1978).
6. Amy Gutman refers to these three interests as equal respect, equality of opportunity, and equal relief from pain ("For and Against Equal Access to Health Care," in *In Search of Equity*, ed. Ronald Bayer, Arthur Caplan, and Norman Daniels [New York: Plenum Press, 1983], p. 51). David Thomasma calls three similar values the religious, political, and medical recognitions of persons' intrinsic value ("Apology," pp. 50–52).
7. See, for example, Thomas E. Hill, Jr., "Servility and Self-Respect," *Monist* 57, no. 1 (January 1973): 87–104.
8. Gene Outka, "Social Justice and Equal Access to Health Care," in *Ethics and Health Policy*, ed. Robert M. Veatch and Roy Branson (Cambridge, Mass.: Ballinger, 1976), pp. 79–98; Plato, *Laws*, vi. 757A: "To unequals, equals become unequal."
9. Outka, "Social Justice and Equal Access," pp. 91–93.
10. See, for example, George Herbert Mead, *Mind, Self, and Society*, ed. Charles Morris (Chicago: University of Chicago Press, 1965), p. 208.
11. Outka, "Social Justice and Equal Access," p. 90. The same point, that the need for health care is the ground for its distribution, is called a "necessary truth" by Bernard Williams, in "The Idea of Equality," in *Philosophy, Politics, and Society*, ed. Peter Laslett and W. G. Runciman (Oxford: Blackwell, 1962), p. 121.
12. Robert M. Veatch, *A Theory of Medical Ethics* (New York: Basic Books, 1981), p. 268.
13. Henry Shue, *Basic Rights* (Princeton, N.J.: Princeton University Press, 1980), pp. 20–34.
14. Eli Ginzberg, "The Grand Illusion of Competition in Health Care," *Journal of the American Medical Association* 8 (April 1983), pp. 1857–1859.

15. Gutman, "For and Against Equal Access," p. 46.
16. Jerry Avorn, "Needs, Wants, Demands, and Interests," in *In Search of Equity*, ed. Ronald Bayer, Arthur Caplan, and Norman Daniels (New York: Plenum Press, 1983), pp. 183–197.
17. David Ozar offers an analysis of basic health care as including what is needed to keep a person from falling below a state of minimal security ("What Should Count as Basic Health Care?" *Theoretical Medicine* 4 [June 1983]: 129–141).
18. Daniel Callahan, "The WHO Definition of Health," *Hastings Center Studies* 1, no. 3 (1973): 77–87.
19. Arthur Caplan, "Values and the Allocation of New Technologies," in *In Search of Equity*, ed. Ronald Bayer, Arthur Caplan, and Norman Daniels (New York: Plenum Press, 1983), pp. 95–124.
20. Charles J. Dougherty, "Prenatal Diagnosis: A Reappraisal," *Linacre Quarterly* 51, no. 2 (May 1984): 128–138. And who would have the right to in utero surgery, the pregnant woman or the fetus? (Charles J. Dougherty, "The Right to Begin Life with a Sound Body and Mind: Fetal Patients and Conflicts with Their Mothers," *University of Detroit Law Review* 63 [Fall 1985]: 89–117).
21. H. Tristram Engelhardt, "Health Care Allocations: Responses to the Unjust, the Unfortunate, and the Undesirable," *Justice and Health Care*, ed. Earl Shelp (Dordrecht, Netherlands: Reidel, 1981), pp. 121–137.
22. Victor Fuchs makes the points that general economic growth has a more favorable impact on the health of the poor than on that of the more well-off and that extensive schooling is the most powerful correlate of good health ("Economics, Health and Post-Industrial Society," *Milbank Memorial Fund Quarterly* 57, no. 2 [Spring 1979]: 157, 159).
23. Outka, "Social Justice and Equal Access," p. 92.
24. Ibid.
25. This is referred to as the "moral hazard" of insurance (but applies to the case of a public health service as well): taking fewer precautions against injury and illness because the medical bill is already covered (Kenneth Arrow, "Uncertainty and the Welfare Economics of Medical Care," *American Economic Review* 53, no. 5 [December 1963]: 941–973).
26. Veatch, *Theory of Medical Ethics*, p. 279.
27. Gutman, "For and Against Equal Access," p. 60; Outka, "Social Justice and Equal Access," pp. 82–85.
28. John L. S. Holloman, Jr., "Access to Health Care," in *Securing Access to Health Care*, ed. President's Commission for the Study of Ethical Problems in Medicine and Biomedical and Behavioral Research (Washington, D.C.: Government Printing Office, 1983), 2: 86–88.
29. Robert M. Veatch, "What Is a 'Just' Health Care Delivery?" in *Ethics and Health Policy*, ed. Robert M. Veatch and Roy Branson (Cambridge, Mass.: Ballinger, 1976), p. 138; Gutman, "For and Against Equal Access," pp. 44, 65.
30. Fried, "Equality and Rights," p. 31. Or worse, would emigration be forbidden? (Robert Nozick, *Anarchy, State, and Utopia* [New York: Basic Books, 1974], pp. 173–174.
31. Gutman, "For and Against Equal Access," pp. 54–55.

5. Libertarianism

1. Immanuel Kant, *Grounding for the Metaphysics of Morals*, trans. James W. Ellington (Indianapolis: Hackett, 1981), pp. 41–45.
2. Robert Nozick, *Anarchy, State, and Utopia* (New York: Basic Books, 1974), pp. 30–33; Wendy Mariner, "Market Theory and Moral Theory in Health Policy," *Theoretical Medicine* 4 (June 1983): 146.
3. Nozick, *Anarchy, State, and Utopia*, p. 26.
4. Ibid., pp. 28–35.
5. Allen Buchanan, "Justice: A Philosophical Review," in *Justice and Health Care*, ed. Earl Shelp (Dordrecht, Nethrlands: Reidel, 1981), p. 14.

6. Ibid., pp. 16–17; Nozick, *Anarchy, State, and Utopia*, p. 149.
7. Robert Sade, "Medical Care as a Right: A Refutation," *New England Journal of Medicine*, 2 December 1971, p. 1289.
8. Nozick, *Anarchy, State, and Utopia*, pp. 26–28.
9. James F. Childress, "A Right to Health Care?" *Journal of Medicine and Philosophy* 4, no. 2 (June 1979): 143.
10. Nozick, *Anarchy, State, and Utopia*, pp. 150–164.
11. Ibid., pp. 175–182; Buchanan, "Justice," p. 11.
12. Nozick, *Anarchy, State, and Utopia*, pp. 152–153.
13. Ibid., p. 231.
14. "Taxation of earnings from labor is on a par with forced labor" (Ibid., p. 169).
15. Ibid., pp. 239–246.
16. Even Nozick admits the redistributive effect of the minimal state's police protection (Ibid., pp. 113–118).
17. John Arras and Andrew Jameton, "Medical Individualism and the Right to Health Care," in *Intervention and Reflection*, 2d ed., ed. Ronald Munson (Belmont, Calif.: Wadsworth, 1983), pp. 544–545.
18. See, for example, Baruch Brody, "Health Care for the Haves and Have-Nots: Toward a Just Basis of Distribution," in *Justice and Health Care*, ed. Earl Shelp (Dordrecht, Netherlands: Reidel, 1981), pp. 156–159, and Joseph M. Boyle, "The Developing Consensus on the Right to Health Care," in *Justice and Health Care*, ed. Margaret Kelly (St. Louis: Catholic Health Association, 1985), p. 81.
19. David Gauthier, "Unequal Need: A Problem of Equity in Access to Health Care," in *Securing Access to Health Care*, ed. President's Commission for the Study of Ethical Problems in Medicine and Biomedical and Behavioral Research (Washington, D.C.: Government Printing Office, 1983), 2: 196–205.
20. Ibid., 2: 197.
21. Bernard Williams, "The Idea of Equality," in *Philosophy, Politics, and Society*, ed. Peter Laslett and W. G. Runciman (Oxford: Blackwell, 1962), pp. 110–131.
22. Sade, "Medical Care as a Right"; 2: p. 1290. Nozick, *Anarchy, State, and Utopia*, p. 234.
23. Gauthier, "Unequal Need," 196.
24. H. Tristram Engelhardt, "Health Care Allocations: Responses to the Unjust, the Unfortunate, and the Undesirable," in *Justice and Health Care*, ed. Earl Shelp (Dordrecht, Netherlands: Reidel, 1981), pp. 126–127.
25. Ibid.
26. This description of a modified libertarian approach is based on Allen Buchanan, "The Right to a Decent Minimum of Health Care," *Philosophy and Public Affairs* 13, no. 1 (Winter 1984): 55–78.
27. Ronald Bayer, "Ethics, Politics, and Access to Health Care: A Critical Analysis of the President's Commission for the Study of Ethical Problems in Medicine and Biomedical and Behavioral Research," *Cardozo Law Review* 6, no. 2 (Winter 1984): 310.
28. President's Commission for the Study of Ethical Problems in Medicine and Biomedical and Behavioral Research, ed., *Securing Access to Health Care* (Washington, D.C., Government Printing Office, 1983), 1: 22, 34.
29. Ibid., 1: 34.
30. Gauthier, "Unequal Need," 2: 197.
31. Michael Walzer, *Spheres of Justice* (New York: Basic Books, 1983), pp. 10–26.
32. Sade, "Medical Care as a Right," p. 1290.
33. Patients can be regarded as co-workers in therapeutic contexts, too. (William Ruddick, "Doctors' Rights and Work," *Journal of Medicine and Philosophy* 4, no. 2 [June 1979]: 198).
34. See, for example, Eli Ginzberg, "Academic Health Centers," *Health Affairs* 4, no. 2 (Summer 1985): 5–21.
35. Robert Proulx Heaney and Charles J. Dougherty, *Research for Health Professionals: Analysis, Design, and Ethics* (Ames, Ia.: Iowa State University Press, 1987), chapters 10–14.

36. "If the principle of rectification of violations of the first two principles yields more than one description of holdings, then some choice must be made as to which of these is to be realized. Perhaps the sort of considerations about distributive justice and equality that I argue against play a legitimate role in *this* subsidiary choice" (Nozick, *Anarchy, State, and Utopia*, p. 153).

37. In the relevant section of the oath, the physician swears: "To hold him who has taught me this art as equal to my parents and to live my life in partnership with him, and if he is in need of money to give him a share of mine, and to regard his offspring as equal to my brothers in male lineage and to teach them this art—if they desire to learn it—without fee and covenant; to give a share of precepts and oral instruction and all the other learning to my sons and to the sons of him who has instructed me and to pupils who have signed the covenant and have taken an oath according to medical law, but to no one else" (Thomas Mappes and Jane Zembaty, eds., *Biomedical Ethics*, 2d ed. New York: McGraw-Hill, 1986), p. 54.

38. Robert M. Veatch, *A Theory of Medical Ethics* (New York: Basic Books, 1981), p. 256. John Iglehart cites these data: in 1980, 36.3 percent of all medical-school applicants' fathers were physicians or other professionals; in 1985, 39 percent. Those from families with incomes exceeding $30,000 annually went up from 41 percent in 1980 to 54 percent in 1985 ("Update: The Uncertain Future of Medical Practice," *Health Affairs* 5 [Fall 1986]: 44).

39. Paul T. Menzel, *Medical Costs, Moral Choices* (New Haven, Conn.: Yale University Press, 1983), pp. 213-229; Norman Daniels, "Understanding Physician Power: A Review of *The Social Transformation of American Medicine*," *Philosophy and Public Affairs* 13, no. 4 (Fall 1984): 347-357.

40. Paul Starr, *The Social Transformation of American Medicine* (New York: Basic Books, 1982), p. 381.

41. Arras and Jameton, "Medical Individualism," p. 546; Dan Brock, "Distribution of Health Care and Individual Liberty," in *Securing Access to Health Care*, ed. President's Commission for the Study of Ethical Problems in Medicine and Biomedical and Behavioral Research (Washington, D.C.: Government Printing Office, 1983), 2: 249-259.

42. Ruddick, "Doctors' Rights and Work," pp. 192-203; Theodore Marmor and Davis Thomas, "Doctors, Politics, and Pay Disputes," in *Political Analysis and American Medical Care*, ed. Theodore Marmor (Cambridge: Cambridge University Press, 1983), pp. 107-130.

43. Veatch, *Theory of Medical Ethics*, p. 268.

44. Ibid., p. 257.

6. Contractarianism

1. Immanuel Kant, *Grounding for the Metaphysics of Morals*, trans. James W. Ellington (Indianapolis: Hackett, 1981), pp. 44–48.

2. For a discussion of the formation of the "I" and the "me" in childhood, see G. H. Mead, *Mind, Self, and Society*, ed. Charles Morris (Chicago: University of Chicago Press, 1965), pp. 173-178.

3. Christopher Lasch, *The Culture of Narcissism* (New York: Norton, 1978), especially pp. 31-52.

4. Ludwig Wittgenstein, *Philosphical Investigations*, trans. G. E. M. Anscombe (New York: Macmillan, 1968), especially pp. 190, 197, 362, 556.

5. This discussion is indebted to John Rawls, *A Theory of Justice* (Cambridge, Mass.: Harvard University Press, 1971).

6. Ibid., pp. 136-142.

7. Ibid., pp. 150-161.

8. Ibid., pp. 60-61.

9. Ibid.

10. Ibid., p. 75.

11. Ibid., pp. 40–45.
12. Norman Daniels, *Just Health Care* (Cambridge: Cambridge University Press, 1985), p. 5.
13. Michael Walzer, *Spheres of Justice* (New York: Basic Books, 1983), p. 79.
14. See, for example, the discussion in Norman Daniels, "Moral Theory and the Plasticity of Persons," *Monist* 62, no. 3 (July, 1979): 265–287.
15. Paul T. Menzel, *Medical Costs, Moral Choices* (New Haven, Conn.: Yale University Press, 1983), pp. 231–235.
16. H. Tristram Engelhardt, "Health Care Allocations: Responses to the Unjust, the Unfortunate, and the Undesirable," in *Justice and Health Care*, ed. Earl Shelp (Dordrecht, ⁻Netherlands: Reidel, 1981), pp. 125–127.
17. Lawrence Stern, "Opportunity and Health Care: Criticisms and Suggestions," *Journal of Medicine and Philosophy* 8 (1983): 339–361, esp. 345.
18. Engelhardt, "Health Care Allocations," p. 130.
19. Robert Nozick, *Anarchy, State, and Utopia* (New York: Basic Books, 1974), pp. 160–164, 183–231.
20. Robert M. Veatch, *A Theory of Medical Ethics* (New York: Basic Books, 1981), pp. 264–265.
21. Rawls, *Theory of Justice*, pp. 3–4, 22–33.
22. Henry Shue, *Basic Rights* (Princeton, N.J.: Princeton University Press, 1980), p. 127.
23. Rawls, *Theory of Justice*, pp. 147–161.
24. David Hume argued that justice is made necessary by natural scarcity (and limited benevolence) and is made possible by the goods derived as a result of social cooperation (*Treatise of Human Nature*, ed. L. A. Selby-Bigge [Oxford: Clarendon Press, 1967], pt. 2, sec 2). According to Charles Fried, the application of the norms of right and wrong are limited to the range in between the trivial and the catastrophic (*Right and Wrong* [Cambridge, Mass.: Harvard University Press, 1978], pp. 10–12).
25. Ronald Green, "Health Care and Justice in Contract Theory Perspective," in *Ethics and Health Policy*, ed. Robert M. Veatch and Roy Branson (Cambridge, Mass.: Ballinger, 1976), p. 118, and "The Priority of Health Care," *Journal of Medicine and Philosophy* 8 (1983): 374.
26. Veatch, *The Theory of Medical Ethics*, pp. 270–276.
27. Green, "Priority of Health Care," p. 378.
28. This is the thrust of Norman Daniels's work in relation to that of John Rawls (*Just Health Care*).
29. Ibid., pp. 26–35.
30. Ibid., p. 54.
31. This view avoids the "social hijacking" of society's resources by those with extravagant desires (Ibid., pp. 36–37).
32. This view avoids the "bottomless pit" of unlimited demand for the satisfaction of needs (Ibid., pp. 52–55).
33. Allen Buchanan, "Justice: A Philosophical Review," in *Justice and Health Care*, ed. Earl Shelp (Dordrecht, Netherlands: Reidel, 1981), p. 19; John Moskop, "Rawlsian Justice and a Human Right to Health Care," *Journal of Medicine and Philosophy* 8 (1983): 335.
34. Daniels, *Just Health Care*, p. 46.
35. Ibid., pp. 103–108.
36. Ibid., p. 54.
37. Ibid., pp. 78–83.
38. Buchanan, "Justice," pp. 18–19.
39. Stern, "Opportunity and Health Care," p. 341.
40. Daniels, *Just Health Care*, pp. 114–139.

7. Plural Foundations

1. Ian Browlie, ed., *Basic Documents on Human Rights* (Oxford: Oxford University Press, 1981); John L. S. Holloman, Jr., "Access to Health Care," in *Securing Access to Health*

Care, ed. President's Commission for the Study of Ethical Problems in Medicine and Biomedical and Behavioral Research (Washington, D.C.: Government Printing Office, 1983), 2: 79–106; Theodore Marmor and James Marone, "The Health Programs of the Kennedy–Johnson Years: An Overview," in *Political Analysis and American Medical Care*, ed. Theodore Marmor (Cambridge: Cambridge University Press, 1983), pp. 131–151.

2. See, for example, Robert Bella et al., *Habits of the Heart* (Berkeley: University of California Press, 1985).

3. An overview of some of the major interest groups among providers is in Stanley Wohl, *The Medical Industrial Complex* (New York: Harmony Books, 1984); for consumers, see James Marone and Theodore Marmor, "Representing Consumer Interests: The Case of American Health Planning," in *Political Analysis and American Medical Care*, ed. Theodore Marmor (Cambridge: Cambridge University Press, 1983), pp. 76–95.

4. William L. Prosser, *The Law of Torts*, 4th ed. (St. Paul, Minn.: West, 1971), pp. 338–350. According to Prosser, United States law "has persistently refused to recognize the moral obligation of common decency and common humanity, to come to the aid of another human being who is in danger, even though the outcome is to cost him his life" (p. 340); he cites as especially "unappetizing" *Handiboe* v. *McCarthy*, 151 S.E. 2nd 905 (1966), in which "it was held that there was no duty whatever to rescue a child licensee drowning in a swimming pool."

5. See, for example, Charles J. Dougherty, "The Right to Health Care: First Aid in the Emergency Room," *Public Law Forum* 4, no. 1 (1984): 101–128.

6. Ibid., p. 123.

7. Specific difficulties in applying this moral obligation to the law include problems of determining a standard of unselfish service to others in need of aid and of making a rule to cover situations in which many persons might fail to rescue one person (Prosser, *Law of Torts*, p. 341).

8. The view that the ultimate premises of morality are given intuitively and cannot be proved is typical of the twentieth-century metaethical school of intuitionism; see, for example, G. E. Moore, *Principia Ethica* (Cambridge: Cambridge University Press, 1968), and H. A. Pritchard, "Does Moral Philosophy Rest on a Mistake?" in *Readings in Ethical Theory*, ed. Wilfrid Sellars and John Hospers (Englewood Cliffs, N.J.: Prentice-Hall, 1970). But it also has deeper roots: intuitive knowledge of first principles is the basis for Aristotle's ethical naturalism (*Nichomachean Ethics*, trans. Martin Ostwald [Indianapolis: Liberal Arts Press, 1962], especially bk. 6, chap. 11 and 12); it is also the framework for Aquinas's famous dictum to "do good and avoid evil" (*Summa Theologica* [New York: Benziger, 1947], I-IIae, question 94).

9. William James, "The Moral Philosopher and the Moral Life," in *Essays in Pragmatism*, ed. Alburey Castell (New York: Hafner Press, 1948), pp. 72–74.

10. Michael Walzer, *Spheres of Justice* New York: Basic Books, 1983), pp. 3–5.

11. See, for example, Ruth Macklin, "Personhood in the Bioethics Literature," *Milbank Memorial Fund Quarterly* 61, no. 1 (Winter 1983): 40.

12. For an elaboration of this sketch, see Richard Rorty, *Philosophy and the Mirror of Nature* (Princeton, N.J.: Princeton University Press, 1982), esp. chap. 8, and Richard Bernstein, *Beyond Objectivism and Relativism* (Philadelphia: University of Pennsylvania Press, 1983), especially pt. 4.

13. Henry Shue argues that security, subsistence, and liberty are the most basic human rights (*Basic Rights* [Princeton, N.J.: Princeton University Press, 1980], pp. 13–34). Subsistence includes the "proper distribution of minimal food, clothing, shelter, and elementary health care" (Ibid., p. 25). According to the contractarian account, most of what Shue calls security and liberty are already covered by the principle of equal greatest liberty.

14. For a discussion of the notion of the core of a right, see Carl Wellman, *A Theory of Rights* (Totowa, N.J.: Rowman and Allanheld, 1985), pp. 81–91.

15. Martin Golding, "The Concept of Rights: An Historical Sketch," in *Bioethics and Human Rights*, ed. Elsie Bandman and Bertram Bandman (Boston: Little, Brown, 1978), p. 46.

16. While acknowledging the role of legal rights based on utility, Jeremy Bentham, for example, excoriated claims for natural moral rights as "nonsense on stilts," designed only to disguise social privilege (*Anarchial Fallacies*, in *Bentham's Political Thought*, ed. Bhikh Parekh [New York: Barnes and Noble, 1973], p. 269).

17. Mark Siegler, "A Right to Health Care: Ambiguity, Professional Responsibility, and Patient Liberty," *Journal of Medicine and Philosophy* 4, no. 2 (June 1979): 148–156.

18. Allen Buchanan calls for distribution on the basis of "enforced beneficience" ("The Right to a Decent Minimum of Health Care," *Philosophy and Public Affairs* 13, no. 1 [Winter 1984]: 231–238).

19. In 1973, for example, a Wisconsin court wrote: "It would shock the public conscience if a person in need of medical emergency aid would be turned down at the door of a hospital having emergency service because that person could not at that moment assure payment for the service" (*Mercy Medical Center of Oshkosh* v. *Winnebago County* 206 N.W. 2nd 198 [1973]).

20. John Moskop, "Rawlsian Justice and a Human Right to Health Care," *Journal of Medicine and Philosophy* 8 (1983): 336–337.

21. David Thomasma, "An Apology for the Value of Human Lives," *Hospital Progress* 63, no. 3 (April 1982): 49.

22. See, generally, Jacques Maritain, *The Rights of Man and Natural Law*, trans. Doris Anson (New York: Scribner, 1943), and A. Passerin d'Entreves, *The Medieval Contribution to Political Thought* (Oxford: Oxford University Press, 1939).

23. Robert Dickman, "Operationalizing Respect for Persons: A Qualitative Aspect of the Right to Health Care," in *In Search of Equity*, ed. Ronald Bayer, Arthur Caplan, and Norman Daniels (New York: Plenum Press, 1983), pp. 170–171.

24. The French Revolution, which was shaped by many of the political and moral traditions that had helped to stimulate the earlier American Revolution, was the occasion for the first modern claim that health care is a natural right of all persons (Laurence B. McCullough, "Rights, Health Care, and Public Policy," *Journal of Medicine and Philosophy* 4, no. 2 [June 1979]: 207).

8. Market Reforms

1. Robert M. Veatch, "Ethical Dilemmas of For-Profit Enterprise in Health Care," in *The New Health Care for Profit*, ed. Bradford H. Gray (Washington, D.C.: National Academy Press, 1983), pp. 132–136; Institute of Medicine, *For-Profit Enterprise in Health Care* (Washington, D.C.: National Academy Press, 1986), especially pp. 182–204.

2. Arnold Relman, "The New Medical–Industrial Complex," *New England Journal of Medicine*, 23 October 1980, pp. 963–965.

3. Samuel Levey and Douglas Hesse, "Bottom Line Health Care?" *New England Journal of Medicine*, 7 March 1985, p. 644.

4. John F. Horty and Daniel M. Mulholland, "Legal Differences Between Investor-Owned and Nonprofit Health Care Institutions," in *The New Health Care for Profit*, ed. Bradford H. Gray (Washington, D.C.: National Academy Press, 1983), pp. 17–34; J. Warren Salmon, "Profit and Health Care: Trends in Corporatization and Proprietization," *International Journal of Health Services* 15, no. 3 (1985): 402. For a discussion of a Utah court decision in which the tax-exempt status of an allegedly not-for-profit hospital was removed because of its for-profit behavior, see Toby Citrin, "Trustees at the Focal Point," *New England Journal of Medicine*, 7 November 1985, pp. 1223–1226.

5. Bruce C. Vladeck, "The Dilemma Between Competition and Community Service," *Inquiry* 22 (Summer 1985): 116–118; Eli Ginzberg, "The Monetarization of Medical Care," *New England Journal of Medicine* 3 May 1984, p. 1162.

6. Arnold Relman, "The Future of Medical Practice," *Health Affairs* 2, no. 2 (Summer 1983): 11. David Hilfiker reports an informal telephone poll made in Washington, D.C., that

"indicates that less than 10 percent of the private physicians in the city have a sliding fee scale or offer the opportunity to defer payments. More than half the physicians even turn down Medicaid patients" ("A Doctor's View of Modern Medicine," *New York Times Magazine*, 23 February 1986, p. 44).

7. Allen R. Dyer, "Ethics, Advertising and the Definition of a Profession," *Journal of Medical Ethics* 11 (June 1985): 72–78. The key Supreme Court case was *Goldfarb* v. *Virginia State Bar* (1975), in which it was held that "learned professions" are not beyond the reach of the Sherman Antitrust Act.

8. Vladeck, "Dilemma Between Competition and Community Service," p. 119. American medical schools increased their number of graduates from 7,081 in 1960 to 16,318 in 1985 (John Iglehart, "Update: The Uncertain Future of Medical Practice," *Health Affairs* 5 [Fall 1986]: 143).

9. David Mechanic, "Cost Containment and the Quality of Medical Care: Rationing Strategies in an Era of Constrained Resources," *Milbank Memorial Fund Quarterly* 63, no. 3 (Summer 1985): 453–474.

10. Richard B. Siegrist, "Wall Street and the For-Profit Hospital Management Companies," in *The New Health Care for Profit*, ed. Bradford H. Gray (Washington, D.C.: National Academy Press, 1983), pp. 35–50.

11. Joseph A. Califano, "The Challenge to the Health Care System: Can the Third Biggest Business Take Care of the Medically Indigent? A Personal Perspective," in *Health Care for the Poor and Elderly: Meeting the Challenge*, ed. Duncan Yaggy (Durham, N.C.: Duke University Press, 1984), pp. 55–57.

12. The failure of the market is detailed in Kenneth Arrow, "Uncertainty and the Welfare Economics of Medical Care," *American Economic Review* 53, no. 5 (December 1963): 941–973; Eli Ginzberg, "The Grand Illusion of Competition in Health Care," *Journal of the American Medical Association*, 8 April 1983, pp. 1857–1859; Peter Singer, "Freedoms and Utilities in the Distribution of Health Care," in *Ethics and Health Policy*, ed. Robert M. Veatch and Roy Branson (Cambridge, Mass.: Ballinger, 1976), pp. 175–193; and Daniel Wikler, "Philosophical Perspectives on Access to Health Care: An Introduction," in *Securing Access to Health Care*, ed. President's Commission for the Study of Ethical Problems in Medicine and Biomedical and Behavioral Research (Washington, D.C.: Government Printing Office, 1983), 2: 109–151.

13. Ginzberg, "Grand Illusion," p. 1858.

14. Mechanic, "Cost Containment and the Quality of Medical Care," p. 471; Paul T. Menzel, *Medical Costs, Moral Choices* (New Haven, Conn.: Yale University Press, 1983), p. 113.

15. Relman, "New Medical–Industrial Complex," p. 966.

16. Veatch, "Ethical Dilemmas," pp. 125–132.

17. Arnold Relman, "Dealing with Conflicts of Interest," *New England Journal of Medicine*, 19 September 1985, pp. 749–751.

18. Ibid.

19. Jon Hamilton reports that the Paracelsus hospital chain in California offers its physicians up to 20 percent of the profit made by discharging patients before they have exhausted their Medicare DRG allotments ("Are Hospitals Saving Money at Your Expense?" *American Health* 5, no. 1 [January–February 1986]: 44).

20. Harold S. Luft cites a study showing that patients of physicians who own X-ray equipment are twice as likely to be X-rayed than patients whose physicians do not own their own equipment ("Economic Incentives and Clinical Decisions," in *The New Health Care for Profit*, ed. Bradford H. Gray [Washington, D.C.: National Academy Press, 1983], p. 111).

21. Veatch, "Ethical Dilemmas," pp. 143–144.

22. Relman, "Dealing with Conflicts of Interest," p. 751. The Institute of Medicine recognizes the potential impact of these conflicts. Its report recommends breaking the link between physicians' decisions about patient care and their financial interests in equipment or personnel, declares it "unethical and unacceptable" for physicians to have economic

interests in health care facilities to which they make referrals, and concludes that bonus incentive plans from organizations in which physicians practice are usually inconsistent with physicians' fiduciary obligations to patients (*For-Profit Enterprise*, pp. 197–198).

23. Singer, "Freedoms and Utilities," pp. 180–181.

24. Veatch, "Ethical Dilemmas," p. 135.

25. See, for example, Paul Starr, *The Social Transformation of American Medicine* (New York: Basic Books, 1982), pp. 420–449.

26. Levey and Hesse, "Bottom Line Health Care?" p. 644.

27. Michigan prohibits physicians from referring patients to any facility in which the practitioners have a financial interest. Pennsylvania prohibits the referral of any patient receiving state medical assistance to any facility in which practitioners have a financial interest. California requires the full disclosure of physicians' financial interests in referrals (Relman, "Dealing with Conflicts of Interest," p. 750).

28. Siegrist, "Wall Street," p. 42; Salmon, "Profit and Health Care," p. 398.

29. Bradford H. Gray and Walter J. McNerney, "For-Profit Enterprise in Health Care," *New England Journal of Medicine*, 5 June 1986, p. 1525, based on Institute of Medicine, *For-Profit Enterprise*; J. Michael Watt et al., "The Comparative Economic Performance of Investor-Owned and Not-for-Profit Hospitals," *New England Journal of Medicine*, 9 January 1986, pp. 89–96; Steven C. Renn et al., "The Effects of Ownership and System Affiliation on the Economic Performance of Hospitals," *Inquiry* 22 (Fall 1985): 219–236; Robert V. Pattison and Hallie Katz, "Investor-Owned and Not-for-Profit Hospitals," *New England Journal of Medicine*, 11 August 1983, pp. 347–353; L. S. Lewin et al., "Investor-Owneds and Nonprofits Differ in Economic Performance," *Hospitals* 55, no. 13 (July 1981): 52–58. In spite of these higher charges, the Institute of Medicine found no evidence of superior (or inferior) quality of care at IOFP ospitals (*For-Profit Enterprise*, p. 189).

30. Watt et al., "Comparative Economic Performance," p. 91. The mean amount for inpatient charges for ancillary services at investor-owned hospitals was found to be 36 percent higher than that at not-for-profit institutions. Ancillary use per admission was 32 percent higher; ancillary use per day, 36 percent higher.

31. Levey and Hesse, "Bottom Line Health Care?" p. 646. For a warning about the implications of advertising surgery in ophthalmology, see Curtis Margo, "Selling Surgery," *New England Journal of Medicine*, 12 June 1986, pp. 1575–1576.

32. Neil Gilbert, *Capitalism and the Welfare State* (New Haven, Conn.: Yale University Press, 1983), pp. 14–19.

33. Institute of Medicine, *For-Profit Enterprise*, p. 194.

34. Lester Thurow, "Medicine Versus Economics," *New England Journal of Medicine*, 5 September 1985, p. 612.

35. Arnold Relman, "Texas Eliminates Dumping," *New England Journal of Medicine*, 27 February 1986, p. 579; Pattison and Katz, "Investor-Owned and Note-for-Profit Hospitals," p. 350. "Health Care for the Poor in 1985" reports that in Texas, for example, for-profits make up 19.1 percent of the state's hospitals, but in 1985 they provided less than 1 percent of the total charity care in the state and accounted for only 2.7 percent of the bad debt (*Clearinghouse Review* 19, no. 9 [January 1986]: 954). Gray and McNerney show that in four states with more than 30 percent of their hospitals run for profit (Florida, Tennessee, Texas, and Virginia), the level of uncompensated care provided by the IOFP hospitals ranged from 3.4 to 3.8 percent of gross patient revenues, compared with 5.5 to 9 percent among these states' not-for-profit hospitals ("For-Profit Enterprise," p. 1526). The Institute of Medicine concluded "that most of the sources of evidence show that for-profit hospitals proportionately provide less uncompensated care than do not-for-profit hospitals, although there are substantial variations in the magnitude of the difference. In several states where for-profit hospitals are numerous, the uncompensated care difference . . . is substantially larger than is shown in national data" (*For-Profit Enterprise*, p. 187).

36. Institute of Medicine, *For-Profit Enterprise*, p. 187; Robert Schiff et al., "Transfers to a Public Hospital," *New England Journal of Medicine*, 27 February 1986, pp. 552–557.

37. Jane Stein, "Industry's New Bottom Line on Health Care Costs: Is Less Better?" *Hastings Center Report* 15, no. 5 (October 1985): 16.
38. "The committee concludes that public policy cannot rely indefinitely on the ability and willingness of health care institutions to generate the funds needed to provide care to those who are unable to pay. Ensuring adequate health care is a societal obligation, and government should make provision for its financing when private coverage is lacking" (Institute of Medicine, *For-Profit Enterprise*, p. 195).
39. Ibid., p. 205. The authors of the supplementary statement were Alexander M. Capron, Eliot Freidson, Arnold S. Relman, Steven A. Schroeder, Katherine Bauer Sommers, Rosemary Stevens, and Daniel Wikler.

9. DRGs, HMOs, and Vouchers

1. James Marone and Andrew Dunham, "Slouching Towards National Health Insurance: The New Health Care Politics," *Yale Journal of Regulation* 2, no. 2 (1985): 263.
2. Judith R. Lave, "Hospital Reimbursement Under Medicare," *Milbank Memorial Fund Quarterly* 62, no. 2 (Spring 1984): 252.
3. "The Soaring Cost of Health Care," in *National Issues Forum* (Dayton, Ohio: Domestic Policy Association, 1984), p. 17; John Iglehart, "Early Experience with Prospective Payment of Hospitals," *New England Journal of Medicine*, 29 May 1986, p. 1461.
4. "Soaring Cost of Health Care," p. 6.
5. "The barber is not the person to ask if you need a haircut" (Jerry Avorn, "Needs, Wants, Demands, and Interests," in *In Search of Equity*, ed. Ronald Bayer, Arthur Caplan, and Norman Daniels [New York: Plenum Press, 1983], p. 195).
6. "Soaring Cost of Health Care," p. 12.
7. Bruce C. Vladeck, "The Dilemma Between Competition and Community Service," *Inquiry* 22 (Summer 1985): 118.
8. Danielle A. Dolenc and Charles J. Dougherty, "DRGs: The Counterrevolution in Financing Health Care," *Hastings Center Report* 15, no. 3 (June 1985): 19–29.
9. John Iglehart, "Where Money and Medicine Meet: A Conversation with HCFA Administrator Carolyne K. Davis," *Health Affairs* 4, no. 2 (Summer 1985): 80.
10. Jane Perkins, "The Effects of Health Cost Containment on the Poor: An Overview," *Clearinghouse Review* 19, no. 8 (December 1985): 836.
11. Lave, "Hospital Reimbursement Under Medicare," p. 260.
12. Perkins, "Effects of Health Care Cost Containment on the Poor," p. 833.
13. Karen Davis et al., "Is Cost Containment Working?" *Health Affairs* 4 (Fall 1985): 82–88.
14. Ibid., p. 82.
15. Bureau of National Affairs, "DRGs: Impact on Employee Relations in the Health Care Industry," *White Collar Report*, 21 August 1985, p. 5.
16. Robert Newcomer, Juanita Wood, and Andrea Sankar, "Medicare Prospective Payment: Anticipated Effect on Hospitals, Other Community Agencies, and Families," *Journal of Health Politics, Policy and Law* 10, no. 2 (Summer 1985): 276.
17. See Chapter 8, note 29.
18. Vladeck, "Dilemma Between Competition and Community Service," p. 120.
19. Ronald Bayer, "Coping with Cost Containment," *Generations* 10, no. 2 (Winter 1985): 41.
20. *Medicare's Prospective Payment System: Knowing Your Rights* (Washington, D.C.: American Association of Retired Persons, 1985), p. 6.
21. U.S. Congress, Senate Special Committee on Aging, *Impact of Medicare's Prospective Payment System on the Quality of Care Received by Medicare Beneficiaries*, staff report, 99th Cong., 1st sess., 1985.
22. Newcomer, Wood, and Sankar, "Medicare Prospective Payment," p. 279.
23. Lester Thurow, "Medicine Versus Economics," *New England Journal of Medicine*, 5 September 1985, p. 612.
24. John Cardinal O'Connor, "The Right to Health Care" (Labor Day Statement of the

Committee on Social Development and World Peace, United States Catholic Conference, 1985), p. 1. Another 7 to 10 million have only partial insurance coverage for a portion of the year (Donald Cohodes, "America: The Home of the Free, the Land of the Uninsured," *Inquiry* 23 [Fall 1986]: 227).

25. "Health Care for the Poor in 1985," *Clearinghouse Review* (January 1986): 953–954. But Congress has mandated that DRG reimbursement be adjusted for this purpose (Iglehart, "Early Experience with Prospective Payment," p. 1463).

26. Lave, "Hospital Reimbursement Under Medicare," p. 257. Hospital suffering from DRG reimbursement is not universal, however. A study conducted by *Business Week* of 892 hospitals in 9 states in 1984 found that after the first year of DRGs, 81 percent of these hospitals realized profits, and the other 19 percent lost money (Iglehart, "Early Experience with Prospective Payment," p. 1462).

27. See Chapter 8, note 35.

28. Perkins, "Effects of Health Care Cost Containment," p. 833.

29. Lave, "Hospital Reimbursement Under Medicare," p. 261.

30. Bayer, "Coping with Cost Containment," p. 42. A survey conducted by the American Medical Association of doctors' experience with DRGs underscores this point. By 1986, the AMA had received 435 written responses representing 8,050 physicians. Sixty-six percent believed that the quality of care had deteriorated. Forty-three percent reported hospital pressures to discharge patients early. Forty-two percent reported a deterioration in hospital administration–physician relations (Iglehart, "Early Experience with Prospective Payment," p. 1464).

31. Jon Hamilton, "Are Hospitals Saving Money at Your Expense?" *American Health* 5, no. 1 (January–February 1986): 44.

32. Senate Committee on Aging, *Impact of Medicare's Prospective Payment System.*

33. Hamilton, "Are Hospitals Saving Money?" p. 43.

34. "Health Care for the Poor," p. 950.

35. Perkins, "Effects of Health Care Cost Containment," p. 833.

36. Ibid.

37. Benson Roe, "Rational Remuneration," *New England Journal of Medicine*, 14 November 1985, p. 1289.

38. Perkins, "Effects of Health Care Cost Containment," p. 836.

39. Marone and Dunham, "Slouching Towards National Health Insurance," p. 281.

40. Davis et al., "Is Cost Containment Working?" p. 88.

41. Jane Stein, "Industry's New Bottom Line on Health Care Costs: Is Less Better?" *Hastings Center Report* 15, no. 5 (October 1985): 17.

42. David Mechanic, "Cost Containment and the Quality of Medical Care: Rationing Strategies in an Era of Constrained Resources," *Milbank Memorial Fund Quarterly* 63, no. 3 (Summer 1985): 461.

43. Harold S. Luft, "Health Maintenance Organizations and the Rationing of Medical Care," in *Securing Access to Health Care*, ed. President's Commission for the Study of Ethical Problems in Medicine and Biomedical and Behavioral Research (Washington, D.C.: Government Printing Office, 1983), 3: 338.

44. Ibid., p. 336.

45. Iglehart, "Where Money and Medicine Meet," pp. 76–79.

46. In essence, this is the approach offered in Alain Enthoven, "Consumer-Choice Health Plan," *New England Journal of Medicine*, 23 and 30 March 1978, pp. 650–658 and 709–720.

47. Avorn, "Needs, Wants, Demands, and Interests," p. 196.

48. Luft, "Health Maintenance Organizations," p. 318.

49. Ibid.

50. Ibid., p. 324.

51. John Arras, "The Neoconservative Health Strategy," in *In Search of Equity*, ed. Ronald Bayer, Arthur Caplan, and Norman Daniels (New York: Plenum Press, 1983), p. 149.

52. Ibid.

53. Luft, "Health Maintenance Organizations," p. 330.

54. Ibid., p. 335.

55. Ibid., pp. 322–323.

56. Theodore Marmor, Richard Boyer, and Julie Greenberg, "Medical Care and Procompetitive Reform," in *Political Analysis and American Medical Care*, ed. Theodore Marmor (Cambridge: Cambridge University Press, 1983), p. 249.

57. Mechanic, "Cost Containment and the Quality of Medical Care," p. 461.

58. Davis et al., "Is Cost Containment Working?" p. 89.

59. Joseph P. Newhouse, et al., "Are Fee-for-Service Costs Increasing Faster than HMO Costs?" *Medical Care* 23, no. 8 (August 1985): 960.

60. Luft, "Health Maintenance Organizations," p. 321.

61. Ibid., p. 339.

62. One possibility, proposed by Clark Havighurst, mandating a minimum number of nonpoor in every HMO to ensure "proxy shopping" for the poor, is explored and criticized by Arras, "Neoconservative Health Strategy," pp. 134–159.

63. Robert M. Veatch, "Ethical Dilemmas of For-Profit Enterprise in Health Care," in *The New Health Care for Profit*, ed. Bradford H. Gray (Washington, D.C.: National Academy Press, 1983), p. 135.

64. This is essentially the view of Milton Friedman and Rose Friedman, *Free to Choose* (New York: Avon, 1979).

65. Loren Lomansky, "Medical Progress and National Health Care," *Philosophy and Public Affairs* 10, no. 1 (Winter 1981): 76.

66. Charles Fried, "Equality and Rights in Medical Care," *Hastings Center Report* 6 (February 1976): 33.

67. Harold S. Luft, "On the Use of Vouchers for Medicare," *Milbank Memorial Fund Quarterly* 62, no. 2 (Spring 1984): 238.

68. Lomansky, "Medical Progress."

69. There may also be a duty to raise the minimum as affluence increases, regardless of recipients' expectations, if one assumes, as Robert Nozick does not, that nature is held in common and that private ownership is merely a practical arrangement to expedite its use for the common good. On this interpretation, the minimum income is taken to be a form of compensation owed to the poor for the privatization of nature and the disproportionately low benefits they derive from this arrangement compared with the nonpoor. Then as general affluence increases, those shut out of it must be compensated to a proportionately greater degree (Baruch Brody, "Health Care for the Haves and Have-Nots: Toward a Just Basis of Distribution," in *Justice and Health Care*, ed. Earl Shelp [Dordrecht, Netherlands: Reidel, 1981], p. 158).

70. Lawrence Stern, "Opportunity and Health Care: Criticisms and Suggestions," *Journal of Medicine and Philosophy* 8 (1983): 339–361.

71. Neil Gilbert, *Capitalism and the Welfare State* (New Haven, Conn.: Yale University Press, 1983), pp. 38–39.

72. Ibid., pp. 36–37.

73. Stern, "Opportunity and Health Care," p. 359.

74. George Sher, "Health Care and the 'Deserving Poor,'" in *Securing Access to Health Care*, ed. President's Commission for the Study of Ethical Problems in Medicine and Biomedical and Behavioral Research (Washington, D.C.: Government Printing Office, 1983), 2: 304.

75. Arras, "Neoconservative Health Strategy," p. 132.

76. Stern, "Opportunity and Health Care," p. 358.

77. Arras, "Neoconservative Health Strategy," p. 136.

78. Marmor, Boyer, and Greenberg, "Medical Care and Procompetitive Reform," p. 245.

79. Ronald Green, "The Priority of Health Care," *Journal of Medicine and Philosophy* 8 (1983): 377.

80. See Chapter 8, note 12.

81. Gilbert, *Capitalism and the Welfare State*, p. 35.
82. Arras, "Neoconservative Health Strategy," p. 147.
83. Ibid., p. 158.
84. Luft, "Use of Vouchers for Medicare," p. 245.
85. Ibid., p. 241.

10. National Health Care Plans

1. Paul Starr, *The Social Transformation of American Medicine* (New York: Basic Books, 1982), pp. 237–243.
2. John F. Dobbyn, *Insurance Law* (St. Paul, Minn.: West, 1981), p. 16.
3. Ronald Bayer and Daniel Callahan, "Medicare Reform: Social and Ethical Perspectives," *Journal of Health Politics, Policy and Law* 10, no. 3 (Fall 1985): 538.
4. Karen Davis, "Medicare Reconsidered," in *Health Care for the Poor and Elderly: Meeting the Challenge*, ed. Duncan Yaggy (Durham, N.C.: Duke University Press, 1984), pp. 77–84.
5. For example, see Lu Ann Aday and Ronald Andersen, "Equity of Access to Medical Care: A Conceptual and Empirical Overview," in *Securing Access to Health Care*, ed. President's Commission for the Study of Ethical Problems in Medicine and Biomedical and Behavioral Research (Washington, D.C.: Government Printing Office, 1983), 3: 19–54.
6. Theodore Marmor and James Marone, "The Health Programs of the Kennedy–Johnson Years: An Overview," in *Political Analysis and American Medical Care*, ed. Theodore Marmor (Cambridge: Cambridge University Press, 1983), pp. 145–146.
7. John Cardinal O'Connor, "The Right to Health Care" (Labor Day Statement of the Committee on Social Development and World Peace, United States Catholic Conference, 1985), p. 3.
8. Karen Davis et al., "Is Cost Containment Working?" *Health Affairs* (Fall 1985): 90.
9. The government primer on Medicare is *Your Medicare Handbook* (Washington, D.C.: Government Printing Office, 1985).
10. Karen Davis, "Access to Health Care: A Matter of Fairness," in *Health Care: How to Improve It and Pay for It* (Washington, D.C.: Center for National Policy, 1985), p. 50.
11. Paul T. Menzel cites congressional testimony by Senator Edward Kennedy to this effect (*Medical Costs, Moral Choices* [New Haven, Conn.: Yale University Press, 1983], p. 7).
12. Bayer and Callahan, "Medicare Reform," p. 534.
13. Ibid., p. 540. But in 1982, 27.4 percent ($191 billion) of all federal outlays went to the elderly, with less than 10 percent of that support based on means-testing of the recipients; that is, it was paid out regardless of other income and financial resources (Ibid., p. 534).
14. Joseph A. Califano, "The Challenge of the Health Care System: Can the Third Biggest Business Take Care of the Medically Indigent? A Personal Perspective," in *Health Care for the Poor and Elderly: Meeting the Challenge*, ed. Duncan Yaggy (Durham, N.C.: Duke University Press, 1984), pp. 51–52.
15. Bayer and Callahan, "Medicare Reform," pp. 537–540.
16. Robert M. Veatch, "What Is a 'Just' Health Care Delivery?" in *Ethics and Health Policy*, ed. Robert M. Veatch and Roy Branson (Cambridge, Mass.: Ballinger, 1976), pp. 142–153.
17. Starr, *Social Transformation of American Medicine*, p. 406.
18. Norman Daniels, *Just Health Care* (Cambridge: Cambridge University Press, 1985), p. 185.
19. Victor Fuchs, "Economics, Health, and Post-Industrial Society," *Milbank Memorial Fund Quarterly* 57, no. 2 (Spring 1979): 170.
20. David Mechanic, "Cost Containment and the Quality of Medical Care: Rationing Strategies in an Era of Constrained Resources," *Milbank Memorial Fund Quarterly* 63, no. 3 (Summer 1985): p. 463.
21. Gail Wilensky, "Solving Uncompensated Hospital Care: Targeting the Indigent and the Uninsured," *Health Affairs* 3, no. 4 (Winter 1984): 54. Wilensky also notes that one-third

of the uninsured are under eighteen; one-third are poor or near poor; and although one-half are employed all or part of the year, they tend to be low-wage earners with low levels of education and, in almost all cases, are unable to obtain insurance through their employers.

22. Menzel, *Medical Costs, Moral Choices*, p. 105.
23. Wilensky, "Solving Uncompensated Hospital Care," p. 52. Those providing the lion's share of this service are teaching hospitals, government hospitals, and, especially, government teaching hospitals. Teaching hospitals account for 27 percent of total hospital charges, but 35 percent of the uncompensated care (charity care plus bad debt); government hospitals have 12 percent of the charges and 16.9 percent of the uncompensated care; and government teaching hospitals account for 6 percent of the total charges, yet 18 percent of all uncompensated care. Those providing less are the voluntary nonteaching hospitals, which account for 53.1 percent of total charges and 41.7 percent of uncompensated care, and investor-owned for-profit hospitals, which have 7.8 percent of the total charges, but only 5.1 percent of the uncompensated care.
24. Kenneth Arrow, "Uncertainty and the Welfare Economics of Medical Care," *American Economic Review* 53, no. 5 (December 1963): 961.
25. Menzel, *Medical Costs, Moral Choices*, p. 104.
26. Methods for developing a severity of illness index are explored in a special issue of *Health Care Financing Review*, 1984 Annual Supplement.
27. Ronald Bayer, Daniel Callahan, Arthur Caplan, and Bruce Jennings, "Toward a New Health Care System: The Challenge of Justice" (A Report from the Hastings Center, 1985), pp. 43–51.
28. Theodore Marmor, Wayne Hoffman, and Thomas Heagy, "National Health Insurance: Some Lessons from the Canadian Experience," in *Political Analysis and American Medical Care*, ed. Theodore Marmor (Cambridge: Cambridge University Press, 1983), p. 179. George Shieber and Jean-Pierre Poullier show that in 1984, 74.4 percent of all Canadian health care spending was public, compared with 41.4 percent of total American health spending ("International Health Care Spending," *Health Affairs* 5 [Fall 1986]: 117.
29. David Himmelstein and Steffie Woolhandler, "Socialized Medicine: A Solution to the Cost Crisis in Health Care in the United States," *International Journal of Health Services* 16 (November 1986): 340–342.
30. Ibid. Between 1970 and 1982, the number of health care administrators in the United States increased by 171 percent, compared with a 48 percent increase in the number of physicians and a 57 percent increase in total health care personnel. Gerald Anderson shows that from 1980 to 1985, the cost of administration had the highest annual percentage increase of any cost in American health care. It averaged a 19.6 percent annual increase during this period, compared, for example, with research, 6.9 percent; hospital costs, 10.7 percent; government public health programs, 11.2 percent; and physician's costs, 12.9 percent ("National Medical Care Spending," *Health Affairs* 5 [Fall 1986]: 126).
31. Himmelstein and Woolhandler, "Socialized Medicine," p. 343.
32. Marmor, Hoffman, and Heagy, "National Health Insurance," pp. 180–181.
33. Ibid., pp. 174–175.
34. Himmelstein and Woolhandler, "Socialized Medicine," pp. 340, 347.
35. Davis, "Access to Health Care," p. 50.
36. For a discussion of catastrophic health insurance plans centered on the problem of long-term nursing-care expenses, see Thomas Rice and Jon Gabel, "Protecting the Elderly Against High Health Care Costs," *Health Affairs* 5 (Fall 1986): 5–21.
37. Theodore R. Marmor, "Rethinking National Health Insurance," in *Political Analysis and American Medical Care*, ed. Theodore R. Marmor (Cambridge: Cambridge University Press, 1983), pp. 197–206. Assuming in 1977 that less than 1 percent of the population had health care expenses over $5,000 in any year, Marmor estimated the cost of the plan described here at $3 billion.
38. "The Soaring Cost of Health Care," in *National Issues Forum* (Dayton, Ohio: Domestic Policy Association, 1984), p. 30.

39. See, for example, Sr. Amata Miller, "The Economic Realities of Universal Access to Health Care," in *Justice and Health Care*, ed. Margaret Kelly (St. Louis: Catholic Health Association, 1985), pp. 118–124, and John Vaisey, *National Health* (Oxford: Robertson, 1984), pp. 105–122.

40. Vaisey, *National Health*, p. 114.

41. Eli Ginzberg, "The Restructuring of U.S. Health Care," *Inquiry* 22 (Fall 1985): 280. Additionally, 59 percent of the American public currently supports national health insurance.

42. The bill is H.R. 2049, introduced into the Ninety-ninth Congress by Representative Ronald V. Dellums. Its contents are described in *Congressional Record*, 12 June 1985, pp. H4221–H4229.

43. Vaisey notes, for example, that London has an excess of acute hospital facilities, but a dearth of health centers for the delivery of primary care (*National Health*, pp. 100–101).

44. For example, the National Center for Health Statistics listed deaths of American children under 1 year of age at 11.2 per 1,000 in 1982, and the National Centers for Disease Control set it at 10.6 in 1985. This would rank the United States about twelfth among nations, with most of Western Europe ahead. Henry J. Aaron and William B. Schwartz put Britain abreast or slightly ahead of the United States on both figures (*The Painful Prescription: Rationing Hospital Care* [Washington, D.C.: Brookings Institution, 1984], p. 12), but Vaisey shows that in the mid- to late 1970s, almost every nation of Western Europe had a longer male life expectancy, at age 45, than did Britain, when the results for England and Wales (28.2 years after age 45) were averaged with those for Scotland (26.5 years) (*National Health*, p. 108). This would mean that the United States ranks behind the bulk of Western Europe. See also Miller, "Economic Realities," p. 123.

45. "Health Care for the Poor in 1985," *Clearinghouse Review* 19, no. 9 (January 1986): 957.

46. Aaron and Schwartz report that under the National Health Service, the British get one-half as many X-rays per capita as Americans, carry out dialysis at less than one-third the American rate, undertake total parenteral feeding one-quarter as often, have only one-sixth the CT-scanning capacity of the United States, perform one-tenth as many coronary-artery surgeries, and have only one-fifth to one-tenth as many intensive-care hospital beds per capita. This last figure is especially significant (*Painful Prescription*, p. 28). In 1982, there were 56,241 ICU beds in the United States, and $27 billion was spent for their use, virtually 1 percent of that year's total gross national product ("Soaring Cost of Health Care," p. 29). Also see Frances H. Miller and Graham A. H. Miller, "*The Painful Prescription*: A Procrustean Perspective?" *New England Journal of Medicine*, 22 May 1986, pp. 1383–1386.

47. Marmor, "Rethinking National Health Insurance," p. 194.

48. Aaron and Schwartz, *Painful Prescription*, p. 6.

49. Ibid., p. 85.

50. Schieber and Poullier, "International Health Care Spending," p. 117.

51. Himmelstein and Woolhandler, "Socialized Medicine," p. 339.

52. Fuchs, "Economics, Health," p. 173.

53. Singer, "Freedom and Utilities in the Distribution of Health Care," in *Ethics and Health Policy*, ed. Robert M. Veatch and Roy Branson (Cambridge, Mass.: Ballinger, 1976), pp. 185–187.

54. Marmor and Marone, "Health Programs of the Kennedy–Johnson Years," p. 145.

55. Vaisey, *National Health*, pp. 101–102.

56. William Ruddick, "Doctors' Rights and Work," *Journal of Medicine and Philosophy* 4, no. 2 (June 1979): 198; Theodore Marmor and Davis Thomas, "Doctors, Politics, and Pay Disputes," in *Political Analysis and American Medical Care*, ed. Theodore Marmor (Cambridge: Cambridge University Press, 1983), pp. 107–30.

57. Norman Daniels, "Why Saying No to Patients in the United States Is So Hard," *New England Journal of Medicine*, 22 May 1986, pp. 1380–1383.

58. This "Kiddicare" suggestion is taken from the work of Theodore Marmor, although he

presents the idea as an insurance program (Marmor, "Rethinking National Health Insurance," pp. 197–205).

59. Ibid., p. 202.

60. "Health Care for the Poor," p. 957. In one Mississippi delta county, for example, the infant mortality rate reaches a staggering 41.7 percent; not 41.7 deaths per 1,000 live births, but 41.7 percent of all births! Assuming the national infant mortality rate to be around 10.5 deaths per 1,000 births, these American infants die at a rate just under 40 times the national average.

Selected Bibliography

Aaron, Henry J., and William B. Schwartz. *The Painful Prescription: Rationing Hospital Care.* Washington, D.C.: Brookings Institution, 1984.

Aday, Lu Ann, and Ronald Andersen. "Equity of Access to Medical Care: A Conceptual and Empirical Overview." In *Securing Access to Health Care,* ed. President's Commission for the Study of Ethical Problems in Medicine and Biomedical and Behavioral Research, 3: 19–54. Washington, D.C.: Government Printing Office, 1983.

Aday, Lu Ann, Ronald Andersen, and Gretchen Fleming. *Health Care in the U.S.: Equitable for Whom?* Beverly Hills, Calif.: Sage, 1980.

Anderson, Gerald. "National Medical Care Spending." *Health Affairs* 5 (Fall 1986): 123–130.

Aristotle, *Nichomachean Ethics,* trans. Martin Ostwald. Indianapolis: Liberal Arts Press, 1962.

Arras, John. "The Neoconservative Health Strategy." In *In Search of Equity,* ed. Ronald Bayer, Arthur Caplan, and Norman Daniels, pp. 125–159. New York: Plenum Press, 1983.

Arras, John, and Andrew Jameton. "Medical Individualism and the Right to Health Care." In *Intervention and Reflection,* 2d ed., ed. Ronald Munson, pp. 541–552. Belmont, Calif.: Wadsworth, 1983.

Arrow, Kenneth. "Uncertainty and the Welfare Economics of Medical Care." *American Economic Review* 53, no. 5 (December 1963): 941–973.

Avorn, Jerry. "Needs, Wants, Demands, and Interests." In *In Search of Equity,* ed. Ronald Bayer, Arthur Caplan, and Norman Daniels, pp. 183–197. New York: Plenum Press, 1983.

Bandman, Elsie, and Bertram Bandman, eds. *Bioethics and Human Rights.* Boston: Little, Brown, 1978.

Bayer, Ronald. "Coping with Cost Containment." *Generations* 10, no. 2 (Winter 1985): 39–42.

———, "Ethics, Politics, and Access to Health Care: A Critical Analysis of the President's Commission for the Study of Ethical Problems in Medicine and Biomedical and Behavioral Research." *Cardozo Law Review* 6, no. 2 (Winter 1984): 303–320.

Bayer, Ronald, and Daniel Callahan. "Medicare Reform: Social and Ethical Perspectives." *Journal of Health Politics, Policy and Law* 10, no. 3 (Fall 1985): 533–547.

Bayer, Ronald, Daniel Callahan, Arthur Caplan, and Bruce Jennings. "Toward a New Health Care System: The Challenge of Justice." A Report from the Hastings Center, mimeo., 1985, pp. 1–54.

Bayer, Ronald, Arthur Caplan, and Norman Daniels, eds. *In Search of Equity*. New York: Plenum Press, 1983.

Beauchamp, Tom L., and James F. Childress. *Principles of Biomedical Ethics*. 2d ed. New York: Oxford University Press, 1983.

Beauchamp, Tom L., and Ruth R. Faden. "The Right to Health and the Right to Health Care." *Journal of Medicine and Philosophy* 4, no. 2 (June 1979): 118–131.

Bell, Nora K. "The Scarcity of Medical Resources: Are There Rights to Health Care?" *Journal of Medicine and Philosophy* 4, no. 2 (June 1979): 158–169.

Berk, Marc, and Gail Wilensky. "Health Care of the Poor Elderly: Supplementing Medicare." *The Gerontologist* 25, no. 3 (June 1985): 311–314.

Bernstein, Richard. *Beyond Objectivism and Relativism*. Philadelphia: University of Pennsylvania Press, 1983.

Blendon, Robert, and David Rogers. "Cutting Medical Costs." *Journal of the American Medical Association*, 14 October 1983, pp. 1880–1884.

Blendon, Robert, Linda Aiken, Howard Freeman, Bradford Kirkman-Liff, and John W. Murphy. "Uncompensated Care by Hospital or Public Insurance for the Poor." *New England Journal of Medicine* 1 May 1986, pp. 1160–1163.

Boyle, Joseph. "The Developing Consensus on the Right to Health Care." In *Justice and Health Care*, ed. Margaret Kelly, pp. 75–90. St. Louis: Catholic Health Association, 1984.

Brock, Dan. "Distribution of Health Care and Individual Liberty." In *Securing Access to Health Care*, ed. President's Commission for the Study of Ethical Problems in Medicine and Biomedical and Behavioral Research, 2: 239–263. Washington, D.C.: Government Printing Office, 1983.

Brody, Baruch. "Health Care for the Haves and Have-Nots: Toward a Just Basis of Distribution." In *Justice and Health Care*, ed. Earl Shelp, pp. 151–159. Dordrecht, Netherlands: Reidel, 1981.

Browlie, Ian, ed. *Basic Documents on Human Rights*. Oxford: Oxford University Press, 1981.

Buchanan, Allen. "Justice: A Philosophical Review." In *Justice and Health Care*, ed. Earl Shelp, pp. 3–21. Dordrecht, Netherlands: Reidel, 1981.

——— . "The Right to a Decent Minimum of Health Care." *Philosophy and Public Affairs* 13, no. 1 (Winter 1984): 55–78.

Califano, Joseph A. "The Challenge to the Health Care System: Can the Third Biggest Business Take Care of the Medically Indigent? A Personal Perspective." In *Health Care for the Poor and Elderly: Meeting the Challenge*, ed. Duncan Yaggy, pp. 45–57. Durham, N.C.: Duke University Press, 1984.

Callahan, Daniel. "Biomedical Progress and the Limits of Human Health." In *Ethics and Health Policy*, ed. Robert M. Veatch and Roy Branson, pp. 157–165. Cambridge, Mass.: Ballinger, 1976.

Caplan, Arthur. "Values and the Allocation of New Technologies." In *In Search of Equity*, ed. Ronald Bayer, Arthur Caplan, and Norman Daniels, pp. 95–124. New York: Plenum Press, 1983.

Carney, Kim. "Cost Containment and Justice." In *Justice and Health Care*, ed. Earl Shelp, pp. 161–178. Dordrecht, Netherlands: Reidel, 1981.

Cassel, Christine. "Doctors and Allocation Decisions: A New Role in the New Medicare." *Journal of Health Politics, Policy and Law* 10, no. 3 (Fall 1985): 549–564.

Childress, James F. "Priorities in the Allocation of Health Care Resources." In *Justice and Health Care*, ed. Earl Shelp, pp. 139–150. Dordrecht, Netherlands: Reidel, 1981.

——— . "A Right to Health Care?" *Journal of Medicine and Philosophy* 4, no. 2 (June 1979): 132–147.

Citrin, Toby. "Trustees at the Focal Point." *New England Journal of Medicine*, 7 November 1985, pp. 1223–1226.

Clark, Phillip. "The Social Allocation of Health Care Resources: Ethical Dilemmas in Age-Group Competition." *The Gerontologist* 25, no. 2 (April 1985): 119–125.

Cohodes, Donald. "America: The Home of the Free, the Land of the Uninsured." *Inquiry* 23 (Fall 1986): 227–235.

Connor, Gerald R. "The Medicaid Program in Transition." In *Securing Access to Health Care*, ed. President's Commission for the Study of Ethical Problems in Medicine and Biomedical and Behavioral Research, 3: 77–103. Washington, D.C.: Government Printing Office, 1983.

Crozier, David A. "Health Status and Medical Care Utilization." *Health Affairs* 3 (Spring 1984): 116.

Cunningham, Robert. *The Healing Mission and the Business Ethic*. Chicago: Pluribus Press, 1982.

Dallek, Geri. "For-Profit Hospitals and the Poor." *Clearinghouse Review* 17, no. 8 (December 1983): 860–867.

Daniels, Norman. "Equity of Access to Health Care: Some Conceptual and Ethical Issues." *Milbank Memorial Fund Quarterly* 60, no. 1 (Winter 1982): 51–81.

———. *Just Health Care*. Cambridge: Cambridge University Press, 1985.

———. "Moral Theory and the Plasticity of Persons." *Monist* 62, no. 3 (July 1979): 265–287.

———. "A Reply to Some Stern Criticisms and a Remark on Health Care Rights." *Journal of Medicine and Philosophy* 8 (1983): 363–317.

———. "Rights to Health Care and Distributive Justice: Programmatic Worries." *Journal of Medicine and Philosophy* 4, no. 2 (June 1979): 174–191.

———. "Understanding Physician Power: A Review of *The Social Transformation of American Medicine*." *Philosophy and Public Affairs* 13, no. 4 (Fall 1984): 347–357.

———. "Why Saying No to Patients in the United States Is So Hard." *New England Journal of Medicine*, 22 May 1986, pp. 1380–1383.

Davis, Edith M., and Michael L. Millman, eds. *Health Care for the Urban Poor*. Totowa, N.J.: Rowman and Allanheld, 1983.

Davis, Karen. "Access to Health Care: A Matter of Fairness." In *Health Care: How to Improve It and Pay for It*, pp. 45–57. Washington, D.C.: Center for National Policy, 1985.

———. "Medicare Reconsidered." In *Health Care for the Poor and Elderly: Meeting the Challenge*, ed. Duncan Yaggy, pp. 77–96. Durham, N.C.: Duke University Press, 1984.

Davis, Karen, Gerald Anderson, Steven Renn, Diane Rowland, Carl Schramm, and Earl Steinberg. "Is Cost Containing Working?" *Health Affairs* 4 (Fall 1985): 81–94.

Davis, Karen, and Diane Rowland. "Uninsured and Underserved: Inequities in Health Care in the U.S." In *Securing Access to Health Care*, ed. President's Commission for the Study of Ethical Problems in Medicine and Biomedical and Behavioral Research, 3: 55–76. Washington, D.C.: Government Printing Office, 1983.

DeCoteau, Jerilyn. "Access of Urban Indians to Health Care." *Clearinghouse Review* 20, no. 4 (Summer 1986): 402–409.

Dickman, Robert. "Operationalizing Respect for Persons: A Qualitative Aspect of the Right to Health Care." In *In Search of Equity*, ed. Ronald Bayer, Arthur Caplan, and Norman Daniels, pp. 161–182. New York: Plenum Press, 1983.

Dolenc, Danielle A, and Charles J. Dougherty. "DRGs: The Counterrevolution in Financing Health Care." *Hastings Center Report* 15, no. 3 (June 1985): 19–29.

Donabedian, Avedis. "The Epidemiology of Quality." *Inquiry* 22 (Fall 1985): 282–292.

Doubilet, Peter, Milton C. Weinstein, and Barbara J. McNeil. "Use and Misuse of the Term 'Cost Effective' in Medicine." *New England Journal of Medicine*, 23 January 1986, pp. 252–256.

Dougherty, Charles J. *Ideal, Fact, and Medicine*. Lanham, Md.: University Press of America, 1985.

———. "The Right to Begin Life with a Sound Body and Mind: Fetal Patients and Conflicts with Their Mothers." *University of Detroit Law Review* 63 (Fall 1985): 89–117.

———. "The Right to Health Care: First Aid in the Emergency Room." *Public Law Forum* 4, no. 1 (1984): 101–128.

Dyer, Allen. "Ethics, Advertising and the Definition of a Profession." *Journal of Medical Ethics* 11, no. 2 (June 1985): 72–78.

Ebert, Robert, and Sarah Brown. "Academic Health Centers." *New England Journal of Medicine*, 19 May 1983, pp. 1200–1208.

Engelhardt, H. Tristram. "Health Care Allocations: Responses to the Unjust, the Unfortunate, and the Undesirable." In *Justice and Health Care*, ed. Earl Shelp, pp. 121–137. Dordrecht, Netherlands: Reidel, 1981.

———. "Rights to Health Care: A Critical Appraisal." *Journal of Medicine and Philosophy* 4, no. 2 (June 1979): 113–117.

Fahey, Charles. "The Infirm Elderly: Their Care and an Agenda for All Segments of Society." *Vital Issues* 31, no. 10 (June 1982): 1–6.

Feder, Judith, Jack Hadley, and Ross Mullner. "Falling Through the Cracks: Poverty, Insurance Coverage, and Hospital Care for the Poor, 1980 and 1982." *Milbank Memorial Fund Quarterly* 62, no. 4 (Fall 1984): 544–566.

Feinberg, Joel. "The Nature and Value of Rights." In *Rights, Justice, and the Bounds of Liberty*, pp. 143–155. Princeton, N.J.: Princeton University Press, 1980, pp. 143–155.

Fried, Charles. "Equality and Rights in Medical Care." *Hastings Center Report* 6 (February 1976): 29–34.

———. "Rights and Health Care—Beyond Equity and Efficiency." *New England Journal of Medicine*, 31 July 1975, pp. 241–245.

Fuchs, Victor. "Economics, Health, and Post-Industrial Society." *Milbank Memorial Fund Quarterly* 57, no. 2 (Spring 1979): 153–183.

Gauthier, David. "Unequal Need: A Problem of Equity in Access to Health Care." In *Securing Access to Health Care*, ed. President's Commission for the Study of Ethical Problems in Medicine and Biomedical and Behavioral Research, 2: 179–205. Washington, D.C.: Government Printing Office, 1983.

Gibbard, Allan. "The Prospective Pareto Principle and Equity of Access to Health Care." In *Securing Access to Health Care*, ed. President's Commission for the Study of Ethical Problems in Medicine and Biomedical and Behavioral Research, 2: 153–178. Washington, D.C.: Government Printing Office, 1983.

Gilbert, Neil. *Capitalism and the Welfare State*. New Haven, Conn.: Yale University Press, 1983.

Ginzberg, Eli. "Academic Health Centers." *Health Affairs* 4, no. 2 (Summer 1985): 5–21.

———. "The Financial Support of Health Care for the Elderly and the Indigent: Economic Perspectives." In *Health Care for the Poor and Elderly: Meeting the Challenge*, ed. Duncan Yaggy, pp. 13–24. Durham, N.C.: Duke University Press, 1984.

———. "The Grand Illusion of Competition in Health Care." *Journal of the American Medical Association*, 8 April 1983, pp. 1857–1859.

———. "The Monetarization of Medical Care." *New England Journal of Medicine*, 3 May 1984, pp. 1162–1165.

———. "The Restructuring of U.S. Health Care." *Inquiry* 22 (Fall 1985): 272–281.

Gray, Bradford H., ed. *The New Health Care for Profit*. Washington, D.C.: National Academy Press, 1983.

Gray, Bradford H., and Walter J. McNerney. "For-Profit Enterprise in Health Care." *New England Journal of Medicine*, 5 June 1986, pp. 1523–1528.

Green, Ronald. "Health Care and Justice in Contract Theory Perspective." In *Ethics and Health Policy*, ed. Robert M. Veatch and Roy Branson, pp. 111–126. Cambridge, Mass.: Ballinger, 1976.

———. "The Priority of Health Care." *Journal of Medicine and Philosophy* 8 (1983): 373–380.

Gutman, Amy. "For and Against Equal Access to Health Care." In *In Search of Equity*, ed. Ronald Bayer, Arthur Caplan, and Norman Daniels, pp. 43–67. New York: Plenum Press, 1983.

Hamilton, Jon. "Are Hospitals Saving Money at Your Expense?" *American Health* 5, no. 1 (January–February 1986): 41–45.

Hayek, F. A. *The Constitution of Liberty*. Chicago: University of Chicago Press, 1960.

"Health Care for the Poor in 1985." *Clearinghouse Review* 19, no. 19 (January 1986): 946–958.

Heaney, Robert Proulx, and Charles J. Dougherty. *Research for Health Professionals: Analysis, Design, and Ethics.* Ames, Iowa: Iowa State University Press, 1987.

Hilfiker, David. "A Doctor's View of Modern Medicine." *New York Times Magazine,* 23 February 1986, pp. 44–47, 58.

Himmelstein, David, and Steffie Woolhandler. "Socialized Medicine: A Solution to the Cost Crisis in Health Care in the United States." *International Journal of Health Services* 15 (November 1986): 339–352.

Hoffman, William. "The Autoworkers' View." *Hastings Center Report* 15, no. 5 (October 1985): 19–20.

Holloman, John L. S., Jr. "Access to Health Care." In *Securing Access to Health Care,* ed. President's Commission for the Study of Ethical Problems in Medicine and Biomedical and Behavioral Research, 2: 79–106. Washington, D.C.: Government Printing Office, 1983.

Horty, John F., and Daniel M. Mulholland. "Legal Differences Between Investor-Owned and Nonprofit Health Care Institutions." In *The New Health Care for Profit,* ed. Bradford H. Gray, pp. 17–34. Washington, D.C.: National Academy Press, 1983.

Iglehart, John. "Early Experience with Prospective Payment of Hospitals." *New England Journal of Medicine,* 29 May 1986, pp. 1460–1464.

––––––. "Growing Attention on Indigent Care May Force Legislators to Act." *Health Progress* (July–August 1985): 8–9.

––––––. "Reducing Residency Opportunities for Graduates of Foreign Medical Schools." *New England Journal of Medicine,* 26 September 1985, pp. 831–836.

––––––. "Update: The Uncertain Future of Medical Practice." *Health Affairs* 5 (Fall 1986): 142–151.

––––––. "Where Money and Medicine Meet: A Conversation with HFCA Administrator Carolyne K. Davis." *Health Affairs* 4, no. 2 (Summer 1985): 72–81.

Institute of Medicine. *For-Profit Enterprise in Health Care.* Washington, D.C.: National Academy Press, 1986.

James, William. "The Moral Philosopher and the Moral Life." In *Essays in Pragmatism,* ed. Alburey Castell, pp. 65–87. New York: Hafner Press, 1948.

Johnson, Dana. "Life, Death, and the Dollar Sign." *Journal of the American Medical Association,* 13 July 1984, pp. 223–224.

Kant, Immanuel. *Grounding for the Metaphysics of Morals,* trans. James W. Ellington. Indianapolis: Hackett, 1981.

Kelly, Margaret, ed. *Justice and Health Care.* St. Louis: Catholic Health Association, 1984.

Lave, Judith. "Hospital Reimbursement Under Medicare." *Milbank Memorial Fund Quarterly* 62, no. 2 (Spring 1984): 251–268.

Levey, Samuel, and Douglas Hesse. "Bottom Line Health Care?" *New England Journal of Medicine,* 7 March 1985, pp. 644–647.

Lomasky, Loren. "Medical Progress and National Health Care." *Philosophy and Public Affairs* 10, no. 1 (Winter 1981): 65–88.

Luft, Harold S. "Economic Incentives and Clinical Decisions." In *The New Health Care for Profit,* ed. Bradford H. Gray, pp. 103–123. Washington, D.C.: National Academy Press, 1983.

––––––. "Health Maintenance Organizations and the Rationing of Medical Care." In *Securing Access to Health Care,* ed. President's Commission for the Study of Ethical Problems in Medicine and Biomedical and Behavioral Research, 3: 313–346. Washington, D.C.: Government Printing Office, 1983.

––––––. "On the Use of Vouchers for Medicare." *Milbank Memorial Fund Quarterly* 62, no. 2 (Spring 1984): 237–250.

Lurie, Nicole et al. "Termination of Medi-Cal Benefits." *New England Journal of Medicine,* 8 May 1986, pp. 1266–1268.

McCullough, Laurence B. "Justice and Health Care: Historical Perspectives and Precedents." In *Justice and Health Care,* ed. Earl Shelp, pp. 51–71. Dordrecht, Netherlands: Reidel, 1981.

———. "Rights, Health Care, and Public Policy." *Journal of Medicine and Philosophy* 4, no. 2 (June 1979): 204–215.

Macklin, Ruth. "Personhood in the Bioethics Literature." *Milbank Memorial Fund Quarterly* 61, no. 1 (Winter 1983): 35–57.

McNerney, Walter J. "Two-Tier System of Health Care." *The Hospital Research and Trust Fund* (1983): 1–7.

Margo, Curtis. "Selling Surgery." *New England Journal of Medicine*, 12 June 1986, pp. 1575–1576.

Mariner, Wendy. "Market Theory and Moral Theory in Health Policy." *Theoretical Medicine* 4 (June 1983): 143–153.

Marmor, Theodore. "Rethinking National Health Insurance." In *Political Analysis and American Medical Care*, ed. Theodore Marmor, pp. 187–206. Cambridge: Cambridge University Press, 1983.

———, ed. *Political Analysis and American Medical Care*. Cambridge: Cambridge University Press, 1983.

Marmor, Theodore, Richard Boyer, and Julie Greenberg. "Medical Care and Procompetitive Reform." In *Political Analysis and American Medical Care*, ed. Theodore Marmor, pp. 239–261. Cambridge: Cambridge University Press, 1983.

Marmor, Theodore, Wayne Hoffman, and Thomas Heagy. "National Health Insurance: Some Lessons from the Canadian Experience." In *Political Analysis and American Medical Care*, ed. Theodore Marmor, pp. 165–186. Cambridge: Cambridge University Press, 1983.

Marmor, Theodore, and James Marone. "The Health Programs of the Kennedy–Johnson Years: An Overview." In *Political Analysis and American Medical Care*, ed. Theodore Marmor, pp. 131–151. Cambridge: Cambridge University Press, 1983.

Marmor, Theodore, and Davis Thomas. "Doctors, Politics and Pay Disputes." In *Political Analysis and American Medical Care*, ed. Theodore Marmor, pp. 107–130. Cambridge: Cambridge University Press, 1983.

Mead, George H. *Mind, Self, and Society*, ed. Charles Morris. Chicago: University of Chicago Press, 1965.

Mechanic, David. "Cost Containment and the Quality of Medical Care: Rationing Strategies in an Era of Constrained Resources." *Milbank Memorial Fund Quarterly* 63, no. 3 (Summer 1985): 453–475.

———. "Rationing Health Care: Public Policy and the Medical Marketplace." *Hastings Center Report* 6 (February 1976): 34–37.

Menzel, Paul T. *Medical Costs, Moral Choices*. New Haven, Conn.: Yale University Press, 1983.

Miller, Sister Amata. "The Economic Realities of Universal Access to Health Care." In *Justice and Health Care*, ed. Margeret Kelly, pp. 109–130. St. Louis: Catholic Health Association, 1985.

Miller, Frances. "Secondary Income from Recommended Treatments: Should Fiduciary Principles Constrain Physician Behavior?" In *The New Health Care for Profit*, ed. Bradford H. Gray, pp. 153–169. Washington, D.C.: National Academy Press, 1983.

Miller, Frances H., and Graham A. H. Miller. "*The Painful Prescription*: A Procrustean Perspective?" *New England Journal of Medicine*, 22 May 1986, pp. 1383–1386.

Mitchell, Janet. "Physician DRGs." *New England Journal of Medicine*, 12 September 1985, pp. 670–675.

Moore, Francis. "Who Should Profit from the Care of Your Illness?" *Harvard Magazine*, November–December, 1985, pp. 45–54.

Morone, James, and Andrew Dunham. "Slouching Towards National Health Insurance: The New Health Care Politics." *Yale Journal on Regulation* 2, no. 2 (1985): 263–291.

Moskop, John. "Rawlsian Justice and a Human Right to Health Care." *Journal of Medicine and Philosophy* 8 (1983): 329–338.

Murphy, Jeffrie. "Rights and Borderline Cases." *Arizona Law Review* 19 (1977): 228–241.

Newcomer, Robert, Juanita Wood, and Andrea Sankar. "Medicare Prospective Payment:

Anticipated Effect on Hospitals, Other Community Agencies, and Families." *Journal of Health Politics, Policy and Law* 10, no. 2 (Summer 1985): 275–282.

Newhouse, Joseph P., William B. Schwartz, Albert P. Williams, and Christina Witsberger. "Are Fee-for-Service Costs Increasing Faster than HMO Costs?" *Medical Care* 23, no. 8 (August 1985): 960–966.

Nietzsche, Friedrich. *Thus Spoke Zarathustra,* in *The Portable Nietzsche,* ed. Walter Kaufmann. New York: Penguin Books, 1983.

No Room in the Marketplace. St. Louis: Catholic Health Association, 1986.

Nozick, Robert. *Anarchy, State, and Utopia.* New York: Basic Books, 1974.

Nutter, Donald. "Access to Care and the Evolution of Corporate, For-Profit Medicine." *New England Journal of Medicine,* October 1984, pp. 917–919.

Outka, Gene. "Social Justice and Equal Access to Health Care." In *Ethics and Health Policy,* ed. Robert M. Veatch and Roy Branson, pp. 79–98. Cambridge, Mass.: Ballinger, 1976.

Ozar, David. "What Should Count as Basic Health Care?" *Theoretical Medicine* 4 (June 1983): 129–141.

Pattison, Robert V., and Hallie Katz. "Investor-Owned and Not-for-Profit Hospitals." *New England Journal of Medicine,* 11 August 1983, pp. 347–353.

Pellegrino, Edmund D. *Humanism and the Physician.* Knoxville: University of Tennessee Press, 1979.

———. "Medical Morality and Medical Economics." *Hastings Center Report* 8, no. 4 (August 1978): 8–12.

Pellegrino, Edmuno D., and David C. Thomasma. *Philosophical Basis of Medical Practice.* New York: Oxford University Press, 1981.

Perkins, Jane. "The Effects of Health Care Cost Containment on the Poor: An Overview." *Clearinghouse Review* 19, no. 8 (December 1985): 831–852.

Plato. *Collected Works,* ed. E. Hamilton and H. Cairns. Princeton, N.J.: Princeton University Press, 1969.

President's Commission for the Study of Ethical Problems in Medicine and Biomedical and Behavioral Research. *Securing Access to Health Care.* Vol. 1, *Report*; Vols. 2 and 3, *Appendices.* Washington, D.C.: Government Printing Office, 1983.

Rawls, John. *A Theory of Justice.* Cambridge, Mass.: Harvard University Press, 1971.

Relman, Arnold. "Dealing with Conflicts of Interest." *New England Journal of Medicine,* 19 September 1985, pp. 749–751.

———. "The Future of Medical Practice." *Health Affairs* 2, no. 2 (Summer 1983): 5–19.

———. "Investor-Owned Hospitals and Health-Care Costs." *New England Journal of Medicine,* 11 August 1983, pp. 370–372.

———. "The New Medical-Industrial Complex." *New England Journal of Medicine,* 23 October 1980, pp. 963–970.

———. "The Power of the Doctors." Review of *The Social Transformation of American Medicine, New York Review of Books,* 29 March 1984, pp. 29–33.

———. "Texas Eliminates Dumping." *New England Journal of Medicine,* 27 February 1986, pp. 578–579.

Renn, Steven et al. "The Effects of Ownership and System Affiliation on the Economic Performance of Hospitals." *Inquiry* 22 (Fall 1985): 219–236.

Rice, Thomas, and Jon Gabel. "Protecting the Elderly Against High Health Care Costs." *Health Affairs* 5 (Fall 1986): 5–21.

Robertson, Marjorie J., and Michael R. Cousineau. "Health Status and Access to Health Services Among the Urban Homeless." *American Journal of Public Health* 76, no. 5 (May 1986): 561–563.

Roe, Benson. "Rational Remuneration." *New England Journal of Medicine,* 14 November 1985, pp. 1286–1289.

Rogers, David. "Providing Medical Care to the Elderly and Poor: A Serious Problem for the Downsizing 80s." In *Health Care for the Poor and Elderly: Meeting the Challenge,* ed. Duncan Yaggy, pp. 3–12. Durham, N.C.: Duke University Press, 1984.

Rorty, Richard. *Philosophy and the Mirror of Nature.* Princeton, N.J.: Princeton University Press, 1979.

Ruddick, William. "Doctors' Rights and Work." *Journal of Medicine and Philosophy* 4, no. 2 (June 1979): 192–203.

Sade, Robert. "Medical Care as a Right: A Refutation." *New England Journal of Medicine,* 2 December 1971, pp. 1288–1292.

Salmon, J. Warren. "Profit and Health Care: Trends in Corporatization and Proprietization." *International Journal of Health Services* 15, no. 3 (1985): 395–418.

Sanders, Charles. "Financial Support of Health Care of the Elderly and the Indigent: Institutions Likely to Be at Risk and Solutions." In *Health Care for the Poor and Elderly: Meeting the Challenge,* ed. Duncan Yaggy, pp. 115–120. Durham, N.C.: Duke University Press, 1984.

Schieber, George, and Jean-Pierre Poullier. "International Health Care Spending." *Health Affairs* 5 (Fall 1986): 111–122.

Schiff, Robert et al. "Transfers to a Public Hospital." *New England Journal of Medicine,* 27 February 1986, pp. 552–557.

Schwartz, Harry. "Access, Equity and Equality in American Medical Care." In *Securing Access to Health Care,* ed. President's Commission for the Study of Ethical Problems in Medicine and Biomedical and Behavioral Research, 2: 67–78. Washington, D.C.: Government Printing Office, 1983.

Shelp, Earl. "Justice: A Moral Test for Health Care and Health Policy." In *Justice and Health Care,* ed. Earl Shelp, pp. 213–229. Dordrecht, Netherlands: Reidel, 1981.

———, ed. *Justice and Health Care.* Dordrecht, Netherlands: Reidel, 1981.

Sher, George. "Health Care and the 'Deserving Poor.'" In *Securing Access to Health Care,* ed. President's Commission for the Study of Ethical Problems in Medicine and Biomedical and Behavioral Research, 2: 293–305. Washington, D.C.: Government Printing Office, 1983.

Shue, Henry. *Basic Rights.* Princeton, N.J.: Princeton University Press, 1980.

Sidel, Victor. "The Right to Health Care: An International Perspective." In *Bioethics and Human Rights,* ed. Elsie Bandman and Bertram Bandman, pp. 341–350. Boston: Little, Brown, 1978.

Siegler, Mark. "A Right to Health Care: Ambiguity, Professional Responsibility, and Patient Liberty." *Journal of Medicine and Philosophy* 4, no. 2 (June 1979): 148–157.

Siegrist, Richard B. "Wall Street and the For-Profit Hospital Management Companies." In *The New Health Care for Profit,* ed. Bradford H. Gray, pp. 35–50. Washington, D.C.: National Academy Press, 1983.

Singer, Peter. "Freedoms and Utilities in the Distribution of Health Care." In *Ethics and Health Policy,* ed. Robert M. Veatch and Roy Branson, pp. 175–193. Cambridge, Mass.: Ballinger, 1976.

Sloan, Frank, and Robert Vraciu. "Investor-Owned and Not-for-Profit Hospitals: Addressing Some Issues." *Health Affairs* 2 (Spring 1983): 25–37.

Starr, Paul. "Medical Care and the Pursuit of Equality in America." In *Securing Access to Health Care,* ed. President's Commission for the Study of Ethical Problems in Medicine and Biomedical and Behavioral Research, 2: 3–22. Washington, D.C.: Government Printing Office, 1983.

———. *The Social Transformation of American Medicine.* New York: Basic Books, 1982.

Stein, Jane. "Industry's New Bottom Line on Health Care Costs: Is Less Better?" *Hastings Center Report* 15, no. 5 (October 1985): 14–18.

Stern, Lawrence. "Opportunity and Health Care: Criticisms and Suggestions." *Journal of Medicine and Philosophy* 8 (1983): 339–361.

Swoap, David. "Beyond DRGs: Shifting the Risk to Providers." *Health Affairs* 3, no. 4 (Winter 1984): 117–121.

Thomasma, David. "An Apology for the Value of Human Lives." *Hospital Progress* 63, no. 3 (April 1982): 49–52, 68.

Thurow, Lester. "Medicine Versus Economics." *New England Journal of Medicine*, 5 September 1985, pp. 611–614.

Townsend, Jessica. "When Investor-Owned Corporations Buy Hospitals: Some Issues and Concerns." In *The New Health Care for Profit*, ed. Bradford H. Gray, pp. 51–72. Washington, D.C.: National Academy Press, 1983.

Updated Report on Access to Health Care for the American People. The Robert Wood Johnson Foundation Special Report, no. 1, 1983.

Vaisey, John. *National Health.* Oxford: Robertson, 1984.

Veatch, Robert M. "Ethical Dilemmas of For-Profit Enterprise in Health Care." In *The New Health Care for Profit*, ed. Bradford H. Gray, pp. 125–152. Washington, D.C.: National Academy Press, 1983.

——— . "Just Social Institutions and the Right to Health Care." *Journal of Medicine and Philosophy* 4, no. 2 (June 1979): 170–173.

——— . *A Theory of Medical Ethics.* New York: Basic Books, 1981.

——— . "What Is a 'Just' Health Care Delivery?" In *Ethics and Health Policy*, ed. Robert M. Veatch and Roy Branson, pp. 127–153. Cambridge, Mass.: Ballinger, 1976.

Veatch, Robert M., and Roy Branson, eds. *Ethics and Health Policy.* Cambridge, Mass.: Ballinger, 1976.

Vladeck, Bruce C. "The Dilemma Between Competition and Community Service." *Inquiry* 22 (Summer 1985): 115–121.

——— . "Equity, Access and the Costs of Health Services." In *Securing Access to Health Care*, ed. President's Commission for the Study of Ethical Problems in Medicine and Biomedical and Behavioral Research, 3: 3–17. Washington, D.C.: Government Printing Office, 1983.

Walzer, Michael. *Spheres of Justice.* New York: Basic Books, 1983.

Watt, J. Michael et al. "The Comparative Economic Performance of Investor-Owned Chains and Not-for-Profit Hospitals." *New England Journal of Medicine*, 9 January 1986, pp. 89–96.

Waxler, Nancy. "The Culture of Medicine Among American Minority Groups." In *Justice and Health Care*, ed. Margaret Kelly, pp. 91–108. St. Louis: Catholic Health Association, 1984.

Weale, Albert. "Statistical Lives and the Principle of Maximum Benefit." *Journal of Medical Ethics* 5, no. 4 (December 1979): 185–195.

Wellman, Carl. *A Theory of Rights.* Totowa, N.J.: Rowman and Allanheld, 1985.

——— . *Welfare Rights.* Totowa, N.J.: Rowman and Littlefield, 1982.

Whitcomb, Michael. "Health Care for the Poor." *New England Journal of Medicine*, 6 November 1986, pp. 1220–1222.

Wikler, Daniel. "Philosophical Perspectives on Access to Health Care: An Introduction." In *Securing Access to Health Care*, ed. President's Commission for the Study of Ethical Problems in Medicine and Biomedical and Behavioral Research, 2: 109–151. Washington, D.C.· Government Printing Office, 1983.

Wilensky, Gail. "Solving Uncompensated Hospital Care: Targeting the Indigent and the Uninsured." *Health Affairs* 3, no. 4 (Winter 1984): 50–62.

Williams, Bernard. "The Idea of Equality." In *Philosophy, Politics, and Society*, ed. Peter Laslett and W. G. Runciman, pp. 110–131. Oxford: Blackwell, 1962.

Wohl, Stanley. *The Medical Industrial Complex.* New York: Harmony Books, 1984.

Wyszewianski, Leon, and Avedis Donabedian. "Equity in the Distribution of Quality of Care." In *Securing Access to Health Care*, ed. President's Commission for the Study of Ethical Problems in Medicine and Biomedical and Behavioral Research, 3: 131–171. Washington, D.C.: Government Printing Office, 1983.

Yaggy, Duncan, ed. *Health Care for the Poor and Elderly: Meeting the Challenge.* Durham, N.C.: Duke University Press, 1984.

Zook, Christopher, and Francis Moore. "High Cost Users of Medical Care." *New England Journal of Medicine*, 1 May 1980, pp. 996–1002.

Index